597

THE SMALL GUIDE TO ALZHEIMER'S DISEASE

THE SMALL GUIDE TO ALZHEIMER'S DISEASE

GARY SMALL, M.D., AND GIGI VORGAN

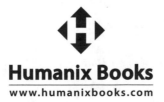

Humanix Books
www.humanixbooks.com

Humanix Books

The Small Guide to Alzheimer's Disease
Copyright © 2020 by Humanix Books
All rights reserved

Humanix Books, P.O. Box 20989, West Palm Beach, FL 33416, USA
www.humanixbooks.com | info@humanixbooks.com

Library of Congress Cataloging-in-Publication Data is available
upon request.

Interior Design: Scribe Inc.

Humanix Books is a division of Humanix Publishing, LLC. Its
trademark, consisting of the words "Humanix Books" is registered
in the Patent and Trademark Office and in other countries.

Disclaimer: The information presented in this book is not specific
medical advice for any individual and should not substitute medical
advice from a health professional. If you have (or think you may have)
a medical problem, speak to your doctor or a health professional
immediately about your risk and possible treatments. Do not engage
in any care of treatment without consulting a medical professional.

ISBN: 978-1-63006-127-2 (Cloth)
ISBN: 978-1-63006-128-9 (E-book)

Printed in the United States of America
10   9   8   7   6   5   4   3   2   1

Contents

Preface

IN MEDICAL SCHOOL, I spent a total of one hour studying Alzheimer's disease. We learned a few facts about memory loss and other symptoms and peeked through a microscope at some brain tissue showing evidence of the disease. At the time, none of my professors or colleagues foresaw the looming epidemic of Alzheimer's on the horizon. Today it is one of the most feared diseases next to cancer. By age 65, the risk for developing Alzheimer's dementia is 10 percent, but by age 85, that risk skyrockets to almost 50 percent—every other person might become affected.

When I became a geriatric psychiatrist, my practice quickly filled with memory-impaired older patients and their worried spouses, adult children, and caregivers hoping for answers but fearing the worst. In *The Small Guide to Alzheimer's Disease*, I describe how doctors assess, diagnose, and treat the disease; provide guidance for caregivers; describe the latest research; and share several stories of how people come face-to-face with Alzheimer's in their families—the challenges they face, the choices they make, and how they can better understand and manage this often overwhelming condition.

Gary Small, M.D.
Los Angeles, CA

CHAPTER 1

Is It Normal Aging or Something Worse?

As you get older three things happen.
The first is your memory goes, and I
can't remember the other two.
　　　　　　　　　　—Sir Norman Wisdom

HELEN, 56, FLIPPED ON the lights in the kitchen, walked straight to the pantry, and stopped dead. *What did I come in here for?* This kind of thing was happening more and more, and it was starting to worry her. Helen poured herself a glass of water and sat down to drink it. She and her friends often joked about getting older and forgetting things, but it didn't seem very funny now. She took another sip of water, then suddenly jumped up and ran to her bathroom, where she'd left the tub filling.

Almost everybody experiences memory lapses from time to time, and age-related memory decline is normal. So why are we all so scared by it? Perhaps because our memory defines who we are. Without our memory we have no past, we cannot plan for the future, and we can't appreciate the present. Another reason memory slips can be so frightening is that they may be an early sign of Alzheimer's disease, one of the scariest diseases we know.

Thanks to healthier lifestyles and medical advances, people are living longer than ever before in human history. In 1950, less than 14 million people reached age 80. By 2000, that number grew to 69 million, and by 2050, it is projected that nearly 380 million people will be 80 years or older. The rub is that this greater life expectancy has also escalated the risk for getting Alzheimer's disease because age is the greatest single risk factor for developing it. In the United States alone, more than 5 million people suffer from Alzheimer's dementia, which gradually robs them of their mental abilities. That number is expected to triple by 2050, making Alzheimer's one of the most feared age-related diseases along with cancer.

WHAT IS ALZHEIMER'S DISEASE?

In 1906, Alois Alzheimer presented to the medical community the first case of what eventually became a disease named after him. He described a woman whose symptoms of confusion began at age 51. In addition to her memory loss, she developed a paranoid psychosis, and her mental clarity rapidly declined until she died at age 55.

When Professor Alzheimer performed an autopsy on her brain, he applied special dyes to the tissue before viewing it under the microscope. He was then able to see, for the first time, the presence of amyloid plaques and tau tangles—abnormal, insoluble protein deposits that had accumulated in brain areas that control memory and thinking.

The medical community found Alzheimer's presentation interesting, but they didn't pay too much attention to his findings. This was probably because it was assumed that Alzheimer's disease was a rare neurodegenerative disorder that only afflicted a few people during middle age. It was thus classified as pre-senile dementia.

Attitudes and attention to the disease changed, however, in 1968, when a group of pathologists published a paper describing autopsy results of a series of older adults who had suffered from senility prior to death. The investigators used the same special dyes that Dr. Alzheimer had applied to the brain tissue of the patient he had presented 60 years earlier. This new study revealed the presence of the same amyloid plaques and tau tangles that were observed in Alzheimer's original pre-senile case. Doctors subsequently talked about early-onset (before age 65) and late-onset (beginning after age 65) Alzheimer's disease rather than pre-senile dementia and senility.

Prior to this new publication, doctors thought that senility was a normal part of aging. If Mom or Grandpa became confused and disoriented, the family would assume that it was just a normal part of old age and there was nothing to be done. The discovery that old-age cognitive symptoms could actually be due to an underlying disease was a wake-up call for researchers. When the scientific world learned of this discovery, doctors and scientists began taking Alzheimer's disease more seriously because it was likely afflicting millions of older adults. This revelation also elicited tremendous fear among the general public who found out about the new epidemic of Alzheimer's disease in older adults.

Regardless of the age at onset, Alzheimer's disease is characterized by a gradual progression of symptoms and the accumulation of amyloid plaques and tau tangles in the brain's frontal (under the forehead), temporal (beneath the temples), and other regions that control thinking and memory. It is the most common type of severe cognitive loss, or dementia, that disrupts patients' ability to care for themselves.

**COMMON PSYCHOLOGICAL REACTIONS
TO AGE-RELATED MEMORY LOSS**

Fear: "I'm losing my mind–I'm going to end up in a nursing home."

Denial: "All my friends are forgetful at my age–there's nothing wrong with me."

Anger: "I get so mad when I can't find the right word."

Self-pity: "Why me? I'm too young to have these problems."

Guilt: "I should have taken better care of myself."

Depression: "I'm nothing without my memory–why should I bother going on like this?"

WHAT'S THE DIFFERENCE BETWEEN ALZHEIMER'S DISEASE AND DEMENTIA?

One of the most frequent questions patients and families ask me involves the difference between Alzheimer's disease and dementia. Briefly, dementia is a cognitive loss that makes a patient dependent on others for care, and Alzheimer's disease is simply the most common type of dementia, accounting for about two-thirds of all dementia cases. Memory is just one aspect of cognition, which refers to several mental skills in addition to memory. These include attention, language ability, reasoning, and visual-spatial functioning.

In part because of the extensive media coverage about Alzheimer's disease, the public has tremendous anxiety about that diagnosis. However, because early interventions can slow down the neurodegeneration of Alzheimer's disease, a diagnosis of dementia from other causes can sometimes have a worse prognosis. For example, a patient who has a severe vascular dementia caused by multiple small strokes may have greater functional impairment than a patient experiencing mild cognitive losses from early-stage Alzheimer's. Also, Alzheimer's disease usually progresses very slowly.

Many different diseases and conditions can cause a dementia syndrome. Dementia from Lewy bodies in the brain has symptoms similar to Alzheimer's disease as well as rigidity and other motor symptoms typical of Parkinson's disease. Frontotemporal dementia primarily affects the frontal and temporal lobes of the brain, causing difficulties in thinking, language, and personality but fewer symptoms of memory loss than in Alzheimer's. In addition to these progressive neurodegenerative diseases, there are some cases where a reversible cause of the dementia is discovered. Anything from drug toxicity to urinary tract infections to depression can lead to cognitive impairments that disrupt a patient's daily functioning.

SYMPTOMS OF DEMENTIA

- Memory loss

- Difficulties in reasoning

- Disorientation, getting lost

- Language difficulties such as word-finding

- Misplacing things

- Mood or personality changes

- Showing less interest or initiative

- Trouble completing familiar tasks like cooking or cleaning

Completely reversible dementias are relatively rare, but I've certainly seen them during the course of my practice. In fact, one of the first patients I saw while training as a geriatric psychiatrist was admitted to the hospital with a working diagnosis of Alzheimer's dementia. During my assessment, I discovered that he had been taking 10 milligrams of Valium (diazepam) every evening for several years. I gradually tapered down his Valium dose, and within a few weeks I had "cured" his dementia.

2
.
Cause

POSSIBLE CAUSES OF DEMENTIA

Although most dementias are chronic and progressive, sometimes a treatable medical cause is uncovered, which reverses some or occasionally all of the symptoms. There are hundreds of different causes of dementia. Below are some of the more common ones and examples.

Possible Cause	Examples
Medical illness	Pneumonia, heart failure, cardiac arrhythmia, thyroid abnormalities, anemia, cancer, liver disease, lung disease, kidney failure, infections, metabolic disturbances, vitamin B12 or folate deficiency, autoimmune disease
Medications	Sedatives, antidepressants, over-the-counter sleep medicines, antihistamines, steroids, pain medicines
Neurodegenerative disorders	Lewy bodies (abnormal brain protein deposits), frontotemporal dementia, Parkinson's disease, normal pressure hydrocephalus (excess brain fluid), vascular disease, Down syndrome
Psychiatric disorders	Depression, anxiety
Other conditions	Head injury, toxic exposures

Because there are so many medical conditions that can cause a dementia, it is important for families and patients to see their doctor if they are concerned about a memory issue. A simple blood test, brain scan, or physical examination can uncover a treatable illness. Early treatment of such illnesses usually yields the best outcome.

Many times, tests reveal that a combination of both a medical illness and progressive neurodegeneration is causing the patient's dementia. However, even in those cases, correcting treatable illnesses like anemias, thyroid abnormalities, or medication side effects can improve the patient's cognitive symptoms to some extent.

THE BRAIN AGES GRADUALLY

Helen, who forgot she left the bathtub filling, and most of her 50-something friends were all noticing memory slips. Usually they joked about it and accepted their forgetfulness as normal for a certain age. But Helen had moments when her concerns were greater, and her symptoms seemed worse when she was under stress or didn't get enough sleep.

With each passing year, an individual's risk for normal memory slips increases. By age 45, memory performance for the average person is significantly worse than their performance was in their mid-20s.

And those objective memory declines correlate with what's known as subjective memory—an individual's self-awareness of their cognitive changes.

What causes these lapses is not entirely clear, but years of scientific inquiry have detailed brain changes that correlate with the symptoms. For example, the amyloid plaques and tau tangles, which Professor Alzheimer described in his original case of the disease, begin to accumulate in the brain decades before people are actually at risk for developing dementia symptoms. Neurotransmitters or brain messengers that permit brain cells to communicate begin to malfunction, and the brain's circulatory system is less effective in transporting oxygen and nutrients from the heart to the brain cells. An aging brain also undergoes wear and tear from head trauma injury, oxidative stress, and heightened inflammation associated with aging.

COMMON SYMPTOMS OF NORMAL BRAIN AGING

- Forgetting names and faces
- Not remembering where you put things
- Failing to recall an appointment or plan
- Forgetting a word or name you should know that is on the tip of your tongue

By middle age, most people start noticing and joking about mild memory slips. But if these cognitive issues progress over the years, then mild cognitive impairment (MCI) may emerge, a transition stage between normal age-related forgetfulness and actual dementia. Most people over 50 have already experienced occasional memory slips, such as blanking on someone's name or the title of a recently read book. If these problems worsen and become more frequent and severe, that's when MCI kicks in.

People experiencing MCI struggle more with their memory. It may take them longer to get out of the house because they're repeatedly searching for misplaced keys or glasses or checking that doors are locked and windows are shut. They may ask the same question more than once during a conversation. Despite these changes, however, these individuals are still able to function independently. They are able to compensate for their increasingly challenging mental abilities. However, when they can no longer compensate for these changes, they may progress to the next stage of brain aging, dementia, or a cognitive deficit that makes them dependent on others for their daily functioning.

Ten percent of people with MCI will develop dementia within a year. This means that in five years, 50 percent of people with MCI will get dementia. Using a brain positron emission tomography (PET) scanning method I developed with my research team at UCLA, it is possible to see into the living brain and watch how it progresses through these stages. As a patient's cognitive symptoms escalate, scans can provide physical evidence of brain shrinkage, buildup of abnormal proteins, decline in cellular function, and other alterations. Using functional MRI scanning, we can observe how neural circuits start to work harder to overcome the encroaching brain disease and compensate for the neurons that have become dysfunctional by recruiting healthy ones to pitch in. Unfortunately, at some point this compensation mechanism breaks down and dementia takes over.

The figure illustrates the slow and steady memory decline that affects nearly everyone if they live long enough. Although age is the biggest risk factor for memory loss, everyone's brain ages at a different rate. In fact, some 90-year-olds have a sharper memory than some 60-year-olds. The transitions between normal aging, MCI, and dementia are very gradual, and what distinguishes dementia from the earlier stages is that patients can no longer live on their own without help.

Memory decline is the main cognitive complaint that most people focus on as they get older, but deterioration in language skills, reasoning, spatial orientation, and concentration can disrupt lives as well. Sometimes patients with MCI experience greater difficulties with decision-making than with memory. Their judgment becomes impaired, and they may

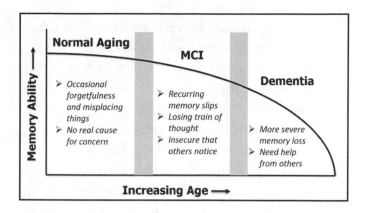

have trouble finding their way around familiar settings. Depression, anxiety, irritability, and other mood changes may emerge, and both cognitive and mood alterations only get worse as MCI progresses to dementia. Personality traits may become altered or exaggerated. For instance, a man who was mildly distrustful of strangers all his life may become paranoid that all strangers are out to get him.

Although normal aging does gradually worsen with time, it remains relatively stable for most people over the years. Despite this stability, some of the physiological changes associated with an aging brain can be observed using brain scanning technologies.

These categories were created to help doctors and scientists communicate and readily describe the degree of cognitive impairment each patient is experiencing. However, the progression of brain aging is slow and subtle in most cases, and the transitions from normal aging to mild cognitive impairment and dementia are not sudden but insidious. The conditions are defined in large part by the patient's ability to function, and that ability will vary from person to person. An executive who has a personal assistant compensating for her cognitive slips may be able to function relatively independently much longer than someone without a personal assistant.

Some people have what's been termed *cognitive reserve.* Their high intelligence allows them to compensate much longer as their brain aging progresses. I've seen several people with cognitive reserve who seem to function quite well—as if they have normal aging—even though their brain scans reveal Alzheimer's disease that appears to be moderate in severity.

DEPRESSION AND ANXIETY WORSEN MEMORY

A 78-year-old retired schoolteacher was brought to the emergency room because of a depressed mood, memory loss, confusion, insomnia, weakness, and agitation. As is typical in emergency room settings, the doctors drew her blood to perform some laboratory tests to search for medical causes of an altered mental state. They also got a brain scan of her head to make sure there wasn't a tumor or brain hemorrhage that could be causing her mental symptoms.

The laboratory tests came back normal, and the brain scan didn't pinpoint any tumors, strokes, or blood clots. The medical team still had several unanswered questions: What is this patient suffering from? Is it Alzheimer's disease? Is it depression? Could it be a combination of the two, or possibly something else entirely? The patient was admitted to the hospital, and over the next week it became clear that she had mild Alzheimer's dementia that was worsened by a depression.

Mood and cognitive symptoms frequently overlap in older adults. Patients with mild cognitive impairment or dementia often experience feelings of anxiety and sadness. Particularly early on in the course of cognitive decline, when patients are aware of their cognitive deficits, they typically experience an emotional reaction to those losses.

Patients with mild memory complaints often tell me how worried they are about their symptoms. Research shows that if patients worry about their symptoms, their memory performance scores will be worse compared to those who do not. Anxiety and other mood changes are distracting and make it difficult to focus attention, which is essential for learning new information and retrieving it later—the basic mental skills needed for effective memory function.

Changes in the brain associated with chronic dementias like Alzheimer's disease can cause imbalances in the brain messengers (i.e., neurotransmitters) that control mood. Once those neurotransmitters decline, the likelihood of mood symptoms increases. Our UCLA group performed PET scans on older patients with major depression, which is a form of depression that is severe enough to require medical intervention. These patients generally experience a persistently depressed mood and loss of pleasure or interest in life as well as disturbed sleep, feelings of guilt, and suicidal thoughts.

In our study, we found that the amyloid plaques and tau tangles that are typical of Alzheimer's disease were also present in the brains of these older patients with major depression. This raises the possibility that symptoms of depression may be a manifestation of Alzheimer's disease in some older patients, especially early in the course of brain neurodegeneration. Other studies have supported the idea that depression can be a risk factor for developing dementia. These issues are critically important because an accurate diagnosis of the underlying condition or conditions is essential for determining the most effective treatment strategy for the symptoms.

Investigators at St. Louis University studied the frequency of mood changes and other behavioral symptoms that occur prior to the diagnosis of dementia as well as after a dementia diagnosis is confirmed. They found that symptoms of depression occurred in approximately half of the patients over 20 months prior to their diagnosis of dementia. Symptoms of anxiety occurred in more than one out of five patients 8 months prior to their diagnosis of dementia. Both depression and anxiety symptoms may continue to develop after the diagnosis of dementia. As the disease progresses, other behavioral disturbances are more likely to emerge, such as agitation, irritability, hallucinations, and aggression.

Often these different syndromes of combined mood and cognitive impairment can be sorted out based on the most prominent symptom, whether it is depression, anxiety, memory loss, or something else. For depression, mood changes are usually present, but physical symptoms are common as well, such as appetite loss, insomnia, and fatigue. However, it can become confusing when patients present with what appears to be a dementia but their condition is actually due to an underlying major depression. The syndrome has been termed *pseudo-dementia*, and patients will complain about memory issues and confusion as well as other symptoms typical of depression, such as sleep disturbances, fatigue, and appetite loss. Interestingly, the patient may not actually feel sad.

DIAGNOSING MAJOR DEPRESSION

To help doctors identify the cluster of symptoms that indicate severe cases of depression that go beyond normal mood fluctuations, they sometimes use a diagnostic mnemonic: *SIG E CAPS*. "SIG" is what doctors write on prescription pad directions and is short for the Latin *signetur*, or "let it be labeled." *E* stands for "energy," and *CAPS* is short for "capsules." So the mnemonic tells us "when to prescribe the energy capsules." Each of the letters stands for one of eight diagnostic features of major depression:

*S*leep decline or increase

*I*nterest loss

*G*uilt feelings

*E*nergy depletion

*C*oncentration difficulties

*A*ppetite change

*P*sychomotor disturbance (e.g., pacing, fidgety, or slowed down)

*S*uicidal thoughts

When people with depression have any four of the *SIG E CAPS* symptoms together, they should see a doctor to determine if they have a major depression that will respond to treatment.

IF IN DOUBT, JUST FIND OUT

Because of fear and anxiety about the possibility of a diagnosis of Alzheimer's disease, many people play down their memory symptoms and deny that they have a problem. It is easy to rationalize since so many people experience forgetfulness as they age. Memory-loss deniers tell themselves that everyone their age has the same forgetfulness they do, so there's probably nothing really wrong.

The danger of waiting while symptoms worsen is that the longer a person waits to seek out help, the further the degree of neurodegeneration, which means that symptomatic treatments may be less effective. The research and common sense indicate that it is easier to protect a healthy brain than to try to repair damage once it becomes extensive.

My advice to people who are concerned about their memory is to have it checked out sooner rather than later. At best, the doctor can reassure the patient that their memory decline is normal for their age. If a diagnosis of mild cognitive impairment or Alzheimer's dementia is made, then the patient can get started early on a treatment. Such treatments will not cure the disease, but they can mitigate the symptoms, delay future cognitive decline, and help the patient live a longer and more fulfilling life despite any cognitive losses.

CHAPTER 2

Seeing the Doctor

*I become faint and nauseous during
even very minor medical procedures,
such as making an appointment by
phone.*

—Dave Barry

MY OFFICE DOOR WAS closed, but I could still hear
my new patient, George, arguing with his wife,
Karen, in the waiting room. Both in their late 60s,
they had been referred to me by their family doctor
because of George's memory problems. I opened the
door and asked them to come in. Karen marched in
first, angry, and sat on the edge of the couch. George
sat beside her and remained silent.

"How can I be of help?" I asked.

"I'm worried about George's memory," Karen said.
"He's forgetting things right and left, and he seems
spaced out half the time. It reminds me of when my

stepfather came down with Alzheimer's disease. He needs help."

I looked to George and asked, "What has it been like for you?"

He shrugged and said, "It's not just me. Everyone I know is becoming forgetful. Even you, Karen."

Karen rolled her eyes. "You see, he's in complete denial. I don't know what to do. It reminds me of my stepfather."

George reached out to comfort her, but Karen moved her arm away.

I said, "I'd like to ask you both some questions and put together a history—"

"Why ask me questions?" Karen snapped. "George is the one with the problem."

George shrugged, and I said, "That's fine, Karen. Perhaps you could step back into the waiting room while I speak with George?"

Karen said, "I'll wait outside."

Once we were alone, George seemed to relax.

"Look, Dr. Small, it's not me, it's Karen who has the problem."

"Oh?"

"Sure, I'm a little forgetful like everyone else I know, but Karen has real memory issues and refuses to admit it."

"When did you start noticing this?"

"She's been gradually losing it for almost two years now. She repeats herself constantly, forgets people's names, and can't find things she just put down. Whenever I try to bring it up, she gets mad and says it's me who has the problem. I don't know what to do."

"So you're saying she is the one in denial?"

"Absolutely. There's no way she would have come with me to see you today if I hadn't said the appointment was for me."

Like Karen, many people in the early stages of cognitive decline are unwilling to face the reality of what it may mean. Fear of memory loss as we age is almost universal because memory is so important to our independence and sense of self. Karen didn't want to accept that her memory was getting worse because she worried that she was developing Alzheimer's like her stepfather did. She felt shame about her increasing forgetfulness and feared that she might eventually become dependent on others for her daily needs. Denial is a common psychological defense mechanism that people use to protect themselves from such uncomfortable feelings but can also delay their discovering what's causing their problem and getting proper treatment. However, it is clearly easier to protect a healthy brain than to try to repair damage once it becomes extensive. Even if someone is suffering from Alzheimer's dementia, research shows that patients who get into treatment early have better outcomes.

And it's not just the patients who slow down the diagnostic and treatment process. Doctors and other healthcare providers often overlook memory problems and other mental symptoms during routine exams. Many healthcare systems and insurance carriers provide disincentives for doctors to care for dementia patients. The time allowed for visits is limited, as are the reimbursements for dementia care. As a result of pushback from patients, families, and the health system, it is estimated that at least half of all patients suffering from Alzheimer's dementia are walking around with it and don't know it.

Although George was not honest with Karen about the reason for their appointment, his ruse worked out for the best. They returned together a week later, and I focused mainly on strategies to improve George's mild, age-related memory slips. Karen got to know me better, felt less defensive about her memory problems, and became more willing to pursue help for herself. She was able to open up about her fading memory, and she finally agreed to let me focus on her issues.

Karen, like many of her peers, used denial to convince herself that her fading memory abilities were a normal part of aging. After all, her friends were all forgetting where they put their keys and glasses too.

Anyone who is living with a family member suffering from Alzheimer's disease knows how patients tend to minimize their symptoms and even hide them from others. This often occurs early in the course of the disease, when patients are aware of the implications of their fading memory abilities but not yet afraid enough to speak up.

NAVIGATING DENIAL

When I first consult with families about a patient's cognitive decline, typically the spouse, siblings, or adult children try to pull me aside in the hallway to talk alone about their fears and concerns. To avoid the awkwardness of these hallway sidebars, I make a point of meeting separately with patients and family members so I can address each of their concerns and offer guidance as to how to engage in these often delicate conversations with their loved one.

Recently, my friend Steve called to talk about his 80-year-old father, Harry, who had been living alone in New Jersey since his wife died six years earlier. Because Steve was busy with his job and family life in Los Angeles, he rarely had time to go back and visit his dad. When his sister Jane called to say that Harry got lost on his walk for the third time, Steve wasn't sure what to do, so he gave me a call.

"I need to get more information, Steve. Does your father have a doctor in New Jersey?"

"Yeah, sure, Gary, but he refuses to go and insists there's nothing wrong with him."

"So I guess he wouldn't see a psychiatrist who I know back there . . ."

"No way. But I'm flying him out here next month for the holidays."

"Maybe you can get your dad to come see me—he already knows me. Maybe I can help figure out what's going on and what the next steps might be."

When Steve picked his father up at the airport, Harry seemed surprised to see him.

"What are you doing here, Steve? Where's Jane?"

"She's home in New Jersey, Dad. You're in Los Angeles. You came to visit me for the holidays."

"I know that—I'm not an idiot!"

"Okay, it's okay. Let's get the car."

Steve called me later. His father was much worse than he'd anticipated. Not only was Harry forgetful; he was ornery and obstinate. There was no chance in hell that Steve was going to get Harry to my office as planned. I had another idea—my wife and I could stop by the house, and I could try to do a casual assessment without Harry even knowing it.

Steve opened the front door and seemed relieved to see us. We went into the den where Harry was watching football.

"The Smalls are here, Dad. You remember them, right?"

Harry looked at us with a total lack of recognition. "Right. How ya doing?"

"Fine. Good to see you." I sat down on the couch and asked, "Who's winning?"

"Winning?"

"The football game?"

"Oh."

I suspected that Harry didn't know who was playing, let alone who was winning.

We sat and chatted during the game. I could see that Harry was having trouble following the conversation, but like so many other patients in the early stages of cognitive impairment, Harry was still pretty good at faking it. He nodded, cheered, and laughed when everyone else was doing it, but I could see he didn't really get the jokes or engage in the conversation.

After the game, we moved to the dining room for dinner, and I sat next to Steve's dad.

"So, Harry, how long are you staying for this trip?"

"Don't know, but it's great having the kids home again."

As we ate our salads, I noted that Harry was having trouble staying oriented and tracking the conversation.

When dinner was served, Harry turned to Steve and said, "Remember when I caught you dressed up in your sister's clothes? You should have seen your face!"

"I was five, Dad."

Harry reached over, grabbed an asparagus spear off my plate, and took a bite. "This is so good."

The more time I spent with Harry, the more convinced I became that he was suffering from a significant cognitive impairment. He could still recall details from years ago, but his memory for recent events was definitely off. In fact, Harry's short-term memory was so bad that it was hard to believe he still lived on his own. Although his symptoms pointed to Alzheimer's dementia, I didn't have enough information to confirm that diagnosis.

I was also concerned about Harry's deteriorating social skills. Eating food off my plate and embarrassing Steve with inappropriate comments suggested a problem in his frontal lobe—the part of the brain that controls judgment and social graces. This kind of behavior can indicate the early stages of frontotemporal dementia, which can often be mistaken for Alzheimer's but has a different brain effect and responds differently to medicines. At the end of the evening, I was convinced that we needed to get Harry in for a brain scan to help pinpoint his diagnosis and get him started on the right treatment.

Unfortunately, getting Harry in for a scan was not the only problem. Steve was having a hard time processing the idea that his father was truly declining mentally. Like many of my patients' family members, Steve was a smart guy who wanted the best for his father, but he hadn't really expected to hear how serious Harry's cognitive decline had become. He was upset, and I can certainly understand that. When my own mother began to forget things and repeat herself over and over, intellectually I knew what was happening, but emotionally I wanted to ignore it. The fact is that denial is a common emotional stage that most people experience when coming to terms with the reality that a loved one may be losing their mental abilities.

CONNECTING WITH A DOCTOR

For many people, overcoming such denial—one way or another—is the first step to getting help. Unfortunately, when patients and their families finally decide they do want help, many are uncertain where to find it. They may not be sure whether a psychiatrist, neurologist, geriatrician, or some other specialist is the best person for them, so they end up seeing numerous specialists and obtaining several unnecessary and repeated evaluations, scans, blood tests, and lumbar punctures. Many times a second opinion is helpful, but too often patients end up with too many conflicting opinions, and rather than focusing on a clear path forward, they can become unsure of who to trust and what to do.

I believe that the best thing to do first is to discuss any memory concerns with a doctor you trust, who is often your primary care physician (PCP). It may be an internist, family practitioner, or any doctor you know and have faith in. Many different specialists and generalists know how to diagnose and treat Alzheimer's disease and related conditions. However, in some circumstances, specific types of specialists are better equipped to deal with the problems at hand.

DOCTORS WHO CARE FOR MEMORY-IMPAIRED PATIENTS

Because of the shortage of neurologists and geriatric psychiatrists, many primary care doctors have developed expertise in diagnosing and treating dementia. Then again, certain clinical situations are best addressed by particular specialists.

- *Primary care physicians.* For typical cases that do not present in unusual ways, internists and family practitioners who have an interest in cognitive problems are able to effectively diagnose and treat patients with dementia.

- *Geriatric psychiatrists.* These specialists are well equipped to care for patients who have symptoms of depression, anxiety, personality change, or psychosis that often develop along with their cognitive symptoms. Geriatric psychiatrists can also be helpful if psychological conflicts emerge among family members.

- *Neurologists.* Any patient experiencing a cognitive decline along with a neurological condition such as Parkinson's disease or Huntington's disease might wish to seek a consultation from a neurologist.

- *Geriatricians.* Patients with multiple medical problems or gait instability, as well as those aged 80 years or older, may benefit from seeing a geriatric internist.

In addition to determining the kind of specialist who might be suitable, it's helpful to come up with a list of the most important qualities you are seeking in a doctor. These may include age, background, clinical style, and other professional qualities. Keep in mind that even if you find a doctor who meets your qualifications, the two of you may not click when you meet in person. That personal connection is important since you will likely have lots of questions for your doctor and you will want to feel comfortable while communicating. Always ask yourself whether this doctor is the kind of person you could trust and who will take your questions seriously. Keep in mind that many doctor/patient relationships strengthen over time as mutual trust builds. However, if your doctor turns out to be unpredictable and inconsistent, it will be hard to develop trust.

One of the best ways to find a doctor is to ask for referrals from people you already trust. If you are not comfortable with your own personal physician but you happen to know someone in the medical field, that person could be an excellent referral source. Friends and relatives who have dealt with patients with cognitive problems themselves can be good referral sources as well. Chances are they went through their own vetting process to find their doctor, and they may be able to enlighten you about who's out there and who might be a good fit for you.

ORGANIZATIONS FOR FINDING A DOCTOR FOR COGNITIVE ISSUES

The websites of the following organizations include links that can guide you to doctors in your area:

- *Alzheimer's Association* (www.alz.com). This national organization provides information on services, programs, publications, and local chapters.

- *Alzheimer's Foundation of America* (www.alzfdn.org). A nonprofit foundation supporting strategies that help lighten the burden and improve the quality of life of Alzheimer's patients and their caregivers.

- *American Academy of Neurology* (www.aan.com). This professional organization advances the art and science of neurology, thereby promoting the best possible care for patients with neurological disorders.

- *American Association for Geriatric Psychiatry* (www .aagponline.org). A professional organization that is dedicated to enhancing the mental health and well-being of older adults through education and research.

- *American Geriatrics Society* (www.americangeriatrics .org). A professional association that provides assistance in identifying local geriatric physician referrals.

- *American Psychiatric Association* (www.psychiatry.org). A medical specialty society that works to ensure that mental disorders are accurately diagnosed and receive effective treatments.

Another important referral source is your local university medical center department of psychiatry, neurology, or medicine, particularly geriatric medicine. Doctors affiliated with reputable academic medical centers are generally accomplished individuals with excellent credentials and experience. Local or national branches of professional societies like the American Psychiatric Association as well as national advocacy groups like the Alzheimer's Association can also be useful referral sources. Members of these groups usually agree to professional and ethical standards set by the organizations, and they often provide continuing education to their members.

WHAT TO EXPECT AT THE DOCTOR'S OFFICE

When patients and their families come to me for help with cognitive issues, I take a systematic approach. I try to assess the clinical issues at hand, but I also need to gain the patient's trust if we are to move forward together with a treatment plan. Educating people at the outset about what to expect is an important first step to building that trust—with both patients and their families. Unless the patient has very mild memory complaints, family members usually accompany them to the first visit.

Following introductions, I explain what I hope to accomplish with them at the initial appointment.

I also ask patients and their family members about their expectations so I can better understand what they want to accomplish. I describe the type of information that I need to obtain in order to understand the patient's particular cognitive problems and plan a treatment strategy.

SUMMARY OF ASSESSMENT PROCEDURES

- Obtain a history of the symptoms from patients, caregivers, and family members. This includes the date of onset of problems, other medical conditions, and any medications being taken.

- Perform a neurological and general physical examination as well as a mental status exam using standardized rating scales, such as the Mini Mental State Examination (MMSE) or the Montréal Cognitive Assessment (MoCA) test.

- Determine the patient's functional abilities and level of independence.

- Draw blood for laboratory testing to assess whether medical illnesses are present.

- Perform a brain scan, such as a magnetic resonance imaging (MRI), a computed tomography (CT), or possibly a position emission tomography (PET) study.

Although I first meet with everyone together, I let them know that I will spend time alone with each of them during the appointment. Explaining this at the beginning of the visit helps minimize any anxious or paranoid feelings that patients or family members may experience when I request to speak with individuals alone. It also makes it easier to perform cognitive testing on the patient without caregivers cueing the patient and biasing the assessment. Further, those individual meetings allow family members to speak more freely about their concerns when the patient is out of earshot.

PREPARING FOR THE APPOINTMENT

Visiting the doctor can be quite an anxiety-provoking experience. This is especially true when people are concerned that the diagnosis may be one that will have a negative prognosis, such as Alzheimer's disease. That anxiety can distract patients and family members to the point that they often forget important questions they wanted to ask during the appointment.

It's a good idea, therefore, to write out your questions in advance of the appointment with the doctor so you are sure to cover all the points that you wish to address. It's also helpful to bring in a summary of the patient's medical history. In order for doctors to summarize the patient's problems, they generally follow a systematic approach. Knowing this system that doctors use to organize their notes (see box) can help you prepare for their needs.

INFORMATION CONTAINED IN DOCTOR'S NOTES

- *Chief complaint.* Main symptom(s) of concern to the patient/family

- *History of present illness.* An account of the timeline and nature of the current illness

- *Past history.* A summary of previous relevant illnesses, both general medical issues and neuropsychiatric conditions

- *Educational and social history.* A review of accomplishments and challenges

- *Risk factors and protective factors.* Smoking, alcohol, head trauma history; exercise, diet, psychological stressors; and other relevant lifestyle habits

- *Review of systems.* A check of different body organs and systems (eyes, lower-body function [i.e., gait], lungs, heart, etc.)

- *Pertinent medical history and medications.* These details sometimes shed light on physical conditions that can impair cognition

- *Physical, neurological, and mental exam results, previous test and scan results.* The doctor's summary of the findings from the evaluation procedures and medical record

- *Impression.* The diagnostic impressions listed by the doctor

- *Treatment plan.* The doctor's itemized plan, including need for more testing, medication interventions, and nonpharmacological strategies

MEDICINES THAT WORSEN MEMORY

It's important to bring a list of all the patient's current medications to the appointment with the doctor. Over the years, patients tend to change doctors or have multiple practitioners caring for them, so taking an inventory of all the medicines can not only be revealing; it can also lead to improved cognitive abilities and overall better care. If the medication regimen is disorganized or complicated, I encourage families to bring the actual medication bottles to the appointment so I can review them systematically with the family. This is very important because so many medications can trigger cognitive symptoms, and sorting out what might be causing side effects or drug interactions can have an important impact on the patient's outcome.

Usually patients with cognitive complaints are older, and as we age we are more likely to take multiple medications. Approximately 10 percent of patients presenting with suspected dementia are experiencing a medication side effect that is contributing to the cognitive decline. Several medicines used to treat psychiatric illnesses, sedating drugs, or narcotic agents can disrupt cognition as well. Histamine H2 receptor antagonists (e.g., famotidine or Pepcid, cimetidine or Tagamet) for stomach problems, cardiac medications such as digoxin and beta-blockers, corticosteroids, nonsteroidal anti-inflammatory agents (e.g., naproxen or Aleve, ibuprofen or Motrin), as well as antibiotics can all cause confusion.

DID YOU KNOW?

Although memory lapses are the most common reason that patients see a doctor for cognitive changes, other symptoms can trigger that initial doctor visit as well. For 23 percent of patients, personality changes lead to an evaluation, while 15 percent complain about difficulties with complicated tasks.

BEWARE OF ANTICHOLINERGIC DRUGS

Many people are not aware of the fact that over-the-counter medicines for allergies (diphenhydramine or Benadryl) or sleep (e.g., Sominex, which also contains diphenhydramine) are anticholinergic. This means that they counter the effects of acetylcholine, a neurotransmitter or brain messenger important for normal memory function. In fact, several of the drugs approved for the treatment of Alzheimer's symptoms are effective because they boost the function of this brain messenger. Drugs with anticholinergic properties have been used to treat many symptoms of medical conditions, such as asthma, chronic obstructive pulmonary disease, diarrhea, epilepsy, gastrointestinal problems, insomnia, motion sickness, overactive bladder or urinary incontinence, Parkinson's disease, psychiatric disorders (depression, psychosis, anxiety), muscle relaxation or anesthesia during surgery, and toxicity of certain poisonings.

Medicines with even mild anticholinergic effects may impair memory function in middle-aged and older adults with minimal age-related cognitive complaints. A recent study published in *JAMA Internal Medicine* showed that prolonged exposure to several kinds of strong anticholinergic drugs is associated with a greater risk for developing dementia. In that study, Dr. Carol Coupland and her colleagues studied hundreds of thousands of people in the United Kingdom and found that prolonged exposure to anticholinergic antidepressants, anti-Parkinson's drugs, antipsychotics, bladder anti-muscarinic drugs, and antiepileptic drugs all increased dementia risk. For older people who used the minimum effective daily dose of a single, strong anticholinergic medication over three years, the investigative team found a nearly 50 percent increased risk for developing dementia within a 10-year period.

People with myasthenia gravis, hyperthyroidism, glaucoma, enlarged prostate, high blood pressure, urinary tract blockage, increased heart rate (tachycardia), heart failure, severe dry mouth, hiatal hernia, severe constipation, liver disease, Alzheimer's disease, or Down syndrome should avoid using these medicines. If you are taking a medication that you think may be exposing you to anticholinergic effects that might be impacting your memory, consult with your doctor to determine if there is an alternative medication you can substitute.

ANTICHOLINERGIC MEDICINES
THAT MAY IMPAIR MEMORY

The following is a list of medicines with known anti-cholinergic properties:

Stronger Effects

Amitriptyline (Elavil)
Atropine
Benztropine (Cogentin)
Chlorpheniramine (e.g., Actifed)
Chlorpromazine (Thorazine)
Clomipramine (Anafranil)
Clozapine (Clozaril)
Cyclobenzaprine (e.g., Flexeril)
Cyproheptadine (Periactin)
Desipramine (Norpramin)
Dexchlorpheniramine
Dicyclomine (Bentyl)
Diphenhydramine (e.g., Advil PM, Benadryl, Nytol, Sominex)
Doxepin (Adapin, Sinequan)
Hydroxyzine (Atarax, Vistaril)
Hyoscyamine (e.g., Anaspaz)
Orphenadrine (Norflex)

Imipramine (Tofranil)
Meclizine (Antivert, Bonine)
Nortriptyline (Pamelor)
Olanzapine (Zyprexa)
Oxybutynin (Ditropan, Oxytrol)
Paroxetine (Brisdelle, Paxil)
Perphenazine (Trilafon)
Prochlorperazine (Compazine)
Promethazine (Phenergan)
Protriptyline (Vivactil)
Pseudoephedrine HCl / Triprolidine HCl (Aprodine)
Scopolamine (Transderm Scop)
Thioridazine (Mellaril)
Tolterodine (Detrol)
Trifluoperazine (Stelazine)
Trimipramine (Surmontil)

Continued

ANTICHOLINERGIC MEDICINES THAT MAY IMPAIR MEMORY (*CONTINUED*)

Milder Effects

Alprazolam (Xanax)	Fluphenazine (Prolixin)
Amantadine (Symmetrel)	Furosemide (Lasix)
Baclofen	Hydrochlorothiazide (e.g., Dyazide)
Carisoprodol (Soma)	Loperamide (Imodium)
Cetirizine (Zyrtec)	Loratadine (Alavert, Claritin)
Cimetidine (Tagamet)	
Clorazepate (Tranxene)	Maprotiline
Codeine	Nifedipine (Adalat, Procardia)
Colchicine	Ranitidine (Zantac)
Digoxin (Lanoxicaps, Lanoxin)	Thiothixene (Navane)
Diphenoxylate (Lomotil)	Tizanidine (Zanaflex)

THE DIAGNOSTIC PROCESS

Obtaining an accurate description of the present illness as well as a past history is critically important to the diagnostic process. For patients with very mild memory complaints, it is possible to obtain a reasonably reliable narrative about the events leading up to the initial appointment. When cognitive deficits are greater, however, it's important to elicit information from family members and caregivers who know the patient well.

Initially, the clinician determines the degree of cognitive impairment, which means an assessment of whether the patient has normal aging, mild cognitive impairment, or dementia. Whether the patient is still functionally independent plays a large part in determining the diagnosis. Several brief, standardized assessment tools can provide a general estimate as to which of these three categories the patient fits into.

The most frequently used cognitive assessment tool is called the Mini-Mental State Examination (MMSE). The MMSE consists of 30 items that assess a range of cognitive skills, including orientation to place, time, and person; ability to focus attention; visual-spatial function; language skills; and short-term memory. A score below 23 is usually consistent with a diagnosis of dementia. However, for patients with a high IQ, cognitive reserve, or high educational achievement, a score above 23 might still be consistent with dementia. For such patients, a more sensitive assessment tool, called the Montréal Cognitive Assessment (MoCA) test, is used. This tool assesses similar cognitive skills as well as executive planning abilities. The MoCA test is available in multiple languages at www.mocatest.org. It provides a score ranging from 0 to 30, and initial studies show that people with normal aging score 27 on average. Those with mild cognitive impairment (MCI) average a score of 22, and patients with dementia average a score of 16.

These brief assessments do not confirm a diagnosis but provide information that complements the other data being collected. Sometimes, however, more extensive cognitive testing through a neuropsychological assessment can be useful. Psychologists known as neuropsychologists with special training in performing more extensive batteries of tests provide these assessments. They usually last several hours and provide greater sensitivity and specificity than a briefer instrument. Neuropsychological testing is particularly helpful when the diagnosis is not straightforward or when the doctor wishes to establish a baseline cognitive profile for future consideration.

The doctor will also perform a physical and neurological exam as well as a mental assessment for depression and other psychological symptoms. This information along with blood tests and brain scans will help differentiate various causes of cognitive problems ranging from Alzheimer's disease to frontotemporal dementia. Very often the nature of symptoms and their time course in developing can be a clue to which neurodegenerative disorder may be the underlying cause.

FEATURES OF DIFFERENT TYPES OF DEMENTIA

Disorder	Clinical Features
Alzheimer's disease	• Gradual onset and progression, initial difficulty remembering recent events
Frontotemporal dementia	• Personality changes, impaired judgment, socially inappropriate behavior
Dementia with Lewy bodies	• Visual hallucinations, movement disorder, apathy
Vascular dementia	• Rapid onset and a series of sudden declines due to repeated small strokes

Determining the type of dementia can have implications for treatment planning. For example, medicines available to stabilize symptoms of Alzheimer's dementia may be ineffective or cause side effects in patients with frontotemporal dementia. Approximately 70 percent of all dementias are due to Alzheimer's disease; however, many patients have multiple causes, such as a combination of vascular disease and Alzheimer's disease.

LABORATORY AND GENETIC TESTING

The doctor will routinely order blood tests to determine if a medical illness might be causing cognitive impairment, and a long list of medical problems can contribute to memory loss. Even if there is an underlying diagnosis of Alzheimer's disease, it is still important to obtain these tests because untreated medical illnesses can worsen dementia from any cause.

RECOMMENDED LABORATORY TESTS FOR ASSESSING COGNITION

Complete blood count

Thyroid function

Vitamin B12 and folate levels

Calcium

Glucose

Electrolytes (sodium, potassium, etc.)

Liver function

Fasting lipid (fat) profile

Sedimentation rate

Urinalysis

Occasionally, the patient has a family history of Alzheimer's disease in multiple generations. In these rare families—representing less than one percent of cases—about half of all relatives develop the disease, usually before age 65. These families have what is called an autosomal dominant inheritance pattern (50 percent of relatives get the disease at about the same age), and a genetic mutation actually causes the disease. The doctor may refer such families to a genetic counselor to determine whether each relative wishes to find out if they have the genetic mutation (either a *presenilin* or *amyloid precursor protein* mutation).

For the vast majority of families, these genetic mutations are not relevant. Instead, a common variation or *allele* may be contributing to a genetic risk for the disease. In the mid-1990s, I collaborated with investigators at Duke University in the discovery of the major known genetic risk for Alzheimer's disease, the appolipoprotein E-4, or APOE-4 allele. Approximately 20 percent of the population carries the APOE-4 allele, which slightly increases risk for developing Alzheimer's disease. However, carrying the APOE-4 allele is neither necessary nor sufficient for developing Alzheimer's disease. Some APOE-4 carriers never get the disease, and many noncarriers do. Therefore, APOE testing is not recommended as a predictive test but is still routinely used in research to determine if genetic-risk status affects treatment outcomes.

DIAGNOSTIC SCANS

Several types of brain scanning technologies are available for the evaluation of cognitive impairment and dementia. The American Academy of Neurology recommends that all patients being assessed for cognitive impairment receive a structural imaging scan, either magnetic resonance imaging (MRI) or computed tomography (CT). The main difference is that MRI scans use magnets and CT scans use X-rays. MRIs provide more detailed information about the brain, but they are very loud and involve lying in a narrow tube, which can make some people feel claustrophobic.

The purpose of such scans is to identify the presence of a tumor, brain hemorrhage, stroke, or some other space-occupying abnormality in the brain that could be contributing to memory loss, although it is relatively rare that treatable abnormalities are revealed on a structural imaging study. Occasionally, one of these scans will show greatly enlarged ventricles (brain areas containing cerebrospinal fluid), which can indicate a condition known as normal pressure hydrocephalus (NPH). If identified early in its course, surgical drainage of the brain fluid may improve the patient's cognitive symptoms.

People often become concerned when they learn that their MRI or CT scan shows general atrophy or shrinkage of the brain, but such atrophy is a normal part of aging and not necessarily dementia. Other times an MRI scan may show white matter hyperintensities, which can be an indication of tiny compromises in brain circulation. However, this too can be a normal finding associated with aging and not necessarily indicative of disease.

In some situations, the doctor may order a functional scan known as positron emission tomography (PET). In these studies, a radioactively labeled form of sugar or glucose (called fluorodeoxyglucose, or FDG) is injected into the patient's arm vein. The FDG is taken up by the brain, and the scanner is able to measure the rate that different brain regions use glucose, the brain's main energy source in nonstarvation states. Because multiple studies have shown that the regional pattern of glucose uptake on these PET scans can differentiate Alzheimer's disease from frontotemporal dementia, Medicare will help pay for these scans. In frontotemporal dementia, the frontal (front part of the brain) and temporal (area beneath the temples) lobes will show less glucose uptake. By contrast, regions in the back part of the brain show less uptake early in the course of Alzheimer's disease.

A PET scan showing Lewy body dementia looks very similar to one showing Alzheimer's disease. In both studies, there is lowered metabolism in the temporal (below the temples) and parietal (behind the temples) brain areas that control thinking and memory. However, in Lewy body dementia, metabolic deficits are also observed in the back part of the brain that controls vision, which is consistent with visual hallucinations that many Lewy body patients experience.

Less often, the doctor may request an electroencephalogram (EEG) or single photon emission computed tomography (SPECT) scan. These procedures can offer helpful information to help clarify the diagnosis, but in general they are less sensitive and less specific than FDG-PET scanning.

Sometimes doctors will order a spinal tap to obtain samples of cerebral spinal fluid to assist with the diagnosis. In Alzheimer's disease, there will be an abnormal ratio of amyloid and tau proteins that can help differentiate that disease from other causes of dementia. However, these lumbar punctures can cause headaches and possible infections and tend to be used less in the United States than in some other countries, particularly in northern Europe.

DISCUSSING THE RESULTS OF THE EVALUATION

Depending on how many procedures are performed, the evaluation process may take more than one or two visits, and it generally provides all the necessary information. When the medical practitioner has all the data in hand, it's time to sit down with the patient and family members to discuss the results.

This discussion takes time, and I would be wary of any doctor who tries to rush through it. Usually patients and family members have lots of questions, so I like to schedule an adequate amount of time for these conversations, and I try to remain sensitive to everyone's concerns. Sometimes a family member will contact me in advance to recommend that I avoid using the word "Alzheimer's," which I have no trouble doing. I'm more concerned about communicating the details of what the family can expect as well as ensuring that the patient is compliant with the recommended treatment.

Of course, no one test makes a diagnosis. It's important to put together the big picture and describe how I made my diagnostic conclusions based on all the available data. During the course of this discussion, I try to touch upon everyone's concerns regarding the prognosis, help them set reasonable expectations, and make clear the treatment options that are available. Once there is clarity on the diagnosis, moving forward with treatment and managing treatment expectations is the next step.

CHAPTER 3

The Latest on Medicines and Supplements

It is easy to get a thousand prescriptions but hard to get one single remedy.

—Chinese proverb

LINDA WAS VERY DISCOURAGED about her husband Ron's condition. After retiring at age 70, he was fine for the first six months, but then his memory slips became more apparent. They went to see a local neurologist who performed a full evaluation, including blood tests, an MRI scan, and even a PET scan. The doctor told them that Ron had Alzheimer's disease and wrote him a prescription for Aricept, a memory medicine they knew about from TV ads.

For three months, Linda tried to be patient, but she hadn't seen any improvement from the Aricept.

Ron was still asking the same questions over and over again, and even though he could still reminisce about the old days, he couldn't remember what he had for dinner the night before.

Linda figured that the medicine wasn't working, so she stopped giving it to him, but things only got worse. Ron started getting lost on his neighborhood walks each morning, and he became more withdrawn. He showed almost no interest in conversing with the kids or helping out around the house.

Linda and Ron made an appointment to see me for a second opinion, and my assistant suggested that Linda bring in all the medicines and supplements Ron was taking. They arrived with a shopping bag full of pill bottles, and it took me a while to go through them. Ron was taking several medicines that are typical for someone in his age group: a statin drug for high cholesterol, a medicine for high blood pressure, another for an enlarged prostate, and an empty bottle labeled donepezil 10 milligrams once a day. I figured that Ron was also having trouble sleeping at night because I found a bottle of an over-the-counter sleep aid, Sominex.

I also found some bottles of supplements, including coenzyme Q10, omega-3 fish oil capsules, vitamin D, vitamin E, and four more with Chinese characters. Linda said they had seen a holistic health specialist who recommended the Chinese concoctions for Ron's memory, but they hadn't worked either. She was getting desperate to find help.

Linda's frustration is typical of many patients and family members who seek medical treatment for a loved one with dementia. They are bombarded with conflicting and confusing information and often feel anxious, helpless, and desperate. Even though Ron had received a reasonable evaluation, the communication between the neurologist and the family was not ideal. I agreed that Ron had Alzheimer's dementia and that the neurologist's recommendation to take donepezil (Aricept) was the accepted standard of care for someone with this diagnosis.

The neurologist, however, did not inform Linda that Ron should stop taking the Sominex because it can worsen memory symptoms. In addition, Linda had unrealistic expectations about the potential benefits of donepezil. She had expected to see cognitive *improvement*, but for many patients, this symptomatic medicine only temporarily *stabilizes* the cognitive symptoms of the disease. And if it is discontinued prematurely, cognitive decline accelerates, as it did in Ron's case.

When families don't see any benefit from standard medical treatment, many then search for alternative interventions, especially supplements. Some of the supplements Ron was taking may have been helpful, but the scientific evidence supporting their effectiveness was limited.

After a couple of visits, Linda and Ron learned about what to expect from a medicine like donepezil. I also helped them understand the limitations of some of the supplements that he was taking. I discontinued his over-the-counter sleep medicine, which led to some immediate improvement in his cognitive abilities. I got him to go back on the donepezil and prescribed a second symptomatic drug for his Alzheimer's dementia symptoms. Ron still experienced some insomnia, which I treated successfully with a supplement called melatonin. After a few months, Ron's cognitive symptoms not only stabilized but improved slightly.

MEDICINES FOR TREATING DEMENTIA SYMPTOMS

After scientists realized that Alzheimer's disease was the most common cause of dementia in late life, research in drug development accelerated. Because many different forms of brain dysfunction contribute to the disease, developing anti-Alzheimer treatments has been complicated. Studies on Alzheimer's brains indicated the presence of several different brain abnormalities, like the accumulation of plaques and tangles, or dysfunction of different types of brain cells or neurons. One particular group of neurons known as the *cholinergic* system showed consistent abnormalities. These cells reside in the base of the brain and produce cholinergic neurotransmitters (i.e., brain messengers). Those cholinergic cells connect to regions of the brain showing deficits in Alzheimer's disease on brain PET scans. These are the same brain regions that control thinking and memory.

Scientists then searched for medicines that could improve memory function by enhancing cholinergic activity in the brain. The strategy for boosting brain cholinergic activity that seemed most effective involved reducing the enzyme that breaks down *acetylcholine*, the relevant neurotransmitter. In 1993, the first cholinesterase inhibitor, tacrine (Cognex), was approved for the treatment of Alzheimer's dementia symptoms. Unfortunately, tacrine was not easy to use. It had to be taken four times a day, and in some patients it caused liver damage, so doctors had to periodically check the patient's blood to detect any emergent liver abnormalities.

In 1997, a newer cholinergic drug, donepezil (Aricept), was approved and soon became the most popular medicine for treating the disease. Donepezil was much easier to use because it only needs to be prescribed once a day, and it doesn't cause the liver side effects that tacrine did. Eventually, two other cholinesterase inhibitors were approved for the treatment of Alzheimer's disease, rivastigmine (Exelon) and galantamine (Razadyne). Because rivastigmine pills caused nausea and vomiting in some patients, a transdermal patch form of the drug, which is gentler on the stomach, was developed and is now available.

In 2003, another drug called memantine (Namenda) received FDA approval in the United

States. Memantine disrupts a different brain receptor known as N-methyl-d-aspartate (NMDA). The drug blocks current flow through channels of NMDA receptors that are broadly involved in brain function. Research has shown that adding memantine to a cholinesterase inhibitor drug provides additional cognitive benefits. All of these drugs have proven benefits for memory, other aspects of cognition, and behavioral disturbances associated with cognitive losses. They have even been shown to improve the patient's general functioning as well as lower the burden that the patient's caregiver experiences.

DRUGS FOR TREATING ALZHEIMER'S SYMPTOMS

- *Aricept (donepezil).* Given orally for mild, moderate, or severe dementia

- *Exelon (rivastigmine).* Often given as a transdermal patch for mild or moderate dementia or dementia associated with Parkinson's disease

- *Namenda (memantine).* Given orally for moderate or severe dementia and often combined with either Aricept or Exelon

- *Namzeric.* A single pill that combines donepezil and memantine

- *Razadyne (galantamine).* Another anticholinergic medicine given orally for mild to moderate dementia

These medicines are called symptomatic treatments because they benefit the patient's symptoms if they are taken continuously. However, they do not reverse the underlying disease process and only offer temporary benefits. Over time, the disease does progress, and patients get worse. Taking these medicines does keep patients at a significantly higher level of functioning longer. A typical patient who starts taking a symptomatic medicine has a good chance of being at the same level of functioning a year later, whereas a patient taking a placebo will show significant cognitive and functional decline after a year. In other words, patients on the medicines are better able to take care of their daily needs (e.g., dressing, bathing, etc.) over time thanks to these medications.

Depending on the level of cognitive and functional impairment, patients with Alzheimer's dementia are categorized as either mild, moderate, or severe. The FDA has approved cholinesterase inhibitors for treating mild to moderate Alzheimer's dementia, and specific cholinesterase inhibitors are indicated for other degrees and forms of dementia. For example, donepezil has also been approved for severe Alzheimer's disease and rivastigmine for dementia associated with Parkinson's disease. Research has demonstrated that cholinesterase inhibitors are helpful in treating dementia with Lewy bodies, vascular dementia, and mixed vascular/Alzheimer's dementia. Results for frontotemporal dementia, however, have been mixed. Memantine is indicated only for moderately to severely demented patients with Alzheimer's disease. The bottom line is that for most forms of dementia (except frontotemporal) these medicines are helpful.

All of these drugs have undergone extensive, double-blind, placebo-controlled clinical trials. This means that one group of patients takes the active drug, while another group takes an inactive placebo, and neither the treating doctors nor the patients know who is getting drug and who is receiving placebo at the time of the study. This kind of study design is necessary to prove that the medication offers benefits above and beyond placebo.

These Alzheimer's disease medicines have been tested in patients with mild cognitive impairment, but the results of the experiments were not convincing enough for the FDA to approve them for MCI. A randomized, placebo-controlled trial in patients with MCI showed that donepezil delayed progression to dementia compared with placebo after one year of treatment. However, no difference between drug and placebo was found after three years of treatment. Sometimes doctors will use a cholinesterase inhibitor to treat MCI. Even though this is considered *off-label* use, some patients with MCI do experience benefits from these medicines.

POTENTIAL BENEFITS OF DEMENTIA MEDICINES

- Stabilization or possible temporary improvement of memory and other cognitive abilities
- Less emergence of behavioral disturbances
- Higher levels of everyday functioning for patients
- Lower caregiver burden

The placebo effect can be substantial but is generally temporary. In fact, the initial studies comparing donepezil to placebo showed a placebo benefit equal to a donepezil benefit for the first six weeks of treatment, but after that point, the placebo-treated patients started to decline, while the donepezil-treated patients showed sustained benefits.

GETTING REALISTIC ABOUT ALZHEIMER'S MEDICINES

Although these medicines do offer significant cognitive benefits, the effects can be subtle, so it is important for families to understand the actual medicine effects and to be realistic about what to expect. I explain that they may not notice any cognitive improvements from the medicine, although a few patients do experience modest subjective improvements in memory. I make sure that I don't "oversell" the medicine and build false hopes of improvement. However, if the patient tolerates the medicine, it is important to remain on the drug because it will stabilize the symptoms and delay further cognitive decline. If doctors don't provide this kind of explanation, patients often stop taking their medicine because their expectations of immediate cognitive improvement are not met, so they think it's not working at all. That was certainly the case for Linda and Ron.

Another problem with patient adherence to medication use occurs later in the course of treatment, when patients do begin to decline. Remember, these medicines do not stop the dementing process and eventually—sometimes after six months, other times after several years—cognitive decline progresses. At this point, many patients and caregivers often assume that the drug is no longer working, so they stop the medication prematurely. However, research shows that if they do stop the medicine at that time, the disease will progress even more rapidly. Anticipating this change from stabilization to gradual decline will lower the likelihood that patients will discontinue their medication prematurely.

A clear explanation of potential side effects is another way to manage patient and caregiver expectations and thus increase adherence. The most common side effects of cholinesterase inhibitors are those affecting the stomach and intestines, such as nausea and diarrhea. Consequently, I recommend that patients take the medicine with a meal and a full glass of water. If the patient is unable to tolerate oral donepezil because of these gastrointestinal side effects, I will switch them to a rivastigmine patch, which rarely causes an upset stomach. However, the patch can cause skin irritation, so it's important that the patch be applied to different areas of the upper body or arms each day. Memantine is well-tolerated by most patients but does have some side effects.

POSSIBLE SIDE EFFECTS OF ANTI-ALZHEIMER'S MEDICINES

Medicine	Side Effects
Cholinesterase inhibitors (donepezil, rivastigmine, galantamine)	Nausea, vomiting, diarrhea, loss of appetite, weight loss, slowed heart rate, dizziness, drowsiness, weakness, trouble sleeping, shakiness (tremor), muscle cramps, vivid dreams
Memantine	Body aches, constipation, headaches, fatigue, weight gain, dizziness

For cholinesterase inhibitors, the initial dose is increased after a month on the lower daily dose (e.g., donepezil: 5 to 10 milligrams; rivastigmine patch: 4.6 to 9.5 milligrams) if the patient tolerates the side effects. Memantine is gradually titrated up from 5 to 20 milligrams using a twice daily dosing, which can eventually be switched to a once daily dose (28 milligrams XR form). For patients who might do better on even higher doses of a cholinesterase inhibitor, those are available too (donepezil 23 milligrams and rivastigmine patch 13.3 milligrams). Of course, side effects are more likely to emerge at higher doses, so the doctor may lower the dose or switch to a different medication if necessary. It is also important to remember that if side effects are mild, the patient may adjust to and eventually tolerate the medicine over time.

TREATMENTS FOR MOOD AND BEHAVIOR PROBLEMS

Many people mistakenly consider Alzheimer's disease and other forms of dementia as strictly cognitive disorders, but depression, agitation, psychosis, anxiety, and other mood disturbances and disruptive behaviors can emerge at any point during the course of these illnesses. Approximately four out of five dementia patients become agitated, and one out of four develops a major depression. Such noncognitive symptoms require assessment and treatment to optimize the patient's clinical course.

Although the FDA has not approved medications to treat these behavioral disturbances specifically in the context of dementia, data from nondemented patients with behavioral symptoms have demonstrated the efficacy of several medication classes, particularly antidepressants for major depression and antipsychotics for symptoms of psychosis. It can be a challenge to prescribe such medicines for patients who already have an underlying cognitive decline, but both research and clinical experience point to their effectiveness in certain situations.

DID YOU KNOW?

Antidepressants are effective in treating several symptoms that may occur in people who are not depressed. The SSRI medicine Prozac (fluoxetine) and some older antidepressants such as Elavil (amitriptyline) have been used to treat pain, and Cymbalta (duloxetine) has been approved for the treatment of fibromyalgia. Trazodone helps some people with insomnia, and Wellbutrin (bupropion) has been approved for smoking cessation.

Patients with dementia and concurrent depression may improve following treatment with antidepressant medications. However, some older antidepressants can worsen memory because they have anticholinergic effects (e.g., amitriptyline or Elavil), so it is best to avoid them and use newer medicines like selective serotonin reuptake inhibitors (SSRIs) such as sertraline (Zoloft) and citalopram (Celexa), which are less likely to impair memory. A meta-analysis, which analyzes the results of many studies, assessed the efficacy of antidepressant treatment in patients with both dementia and depression. Response and remission rates for depression were significantly greater for the pooled antidepressant group than for the group that received a placebo. Other studies suggest that SSRI antidepressants may also reduce agitation observed in patients with dementia.

Antipsychotic drugs sometimes diminish psychotic symptoms (e.g., hallucinations, delusions) and agitation in patients with dementia, but the degree of their effect is modest, and they can pose significant side effects. Older medicines like haloperidol (Haldol) may cause parkinsonian symptoms (tremors, stiffness, slowed body movements), and other older medicines like chlorpromazine (Thorazine) cause sedation, low blood pressure when standing up (postural hypotension), and memory impairment from anticholinergic effects. Less often, patients can develop tardive dyskinesia (a neurological disorder characterized by involuntary movements of the face and jaw).

Newer atypical antipsychotic drugs, such as quetiapine (Seroquel), risperidone (Risperdol), olanzapine

(Zyprexa), and aripiprazole (Abilify) can cause other adverse effects, including metabolic syndrome (a cluster of four conditions—increased blood pressure, high blood sugar, excess body fat around the waist, and abnormal cholesterol or triglyceride levels—which increases the risk of heart disease, stroke, and diabetes). They also heighten the risk for heart arrhythmias. Together, such side effects increase mortality rates in older patients with dementia who take antipsychotic medicines. This prompted the FDA to issue black box warnings on these medicines. Doctors, therefore, use them in low doses for short periods and only when necessary.

Anti-anxiety and anticonvulsant medicines have also been used and studied for the treatment of agitation, but minimal scientific evidence supports their use in this setting, and they, too, have undesirable side effects. Their sedating effects may worsen symptoms of confusion, memory impairment, and gait instability. In addition, taking benzodiazepines (e.g., diazepam [Valium], lorazepam [Ativan]) over long periods of time has been associated with an increased risk for developing dementia.

Most people are unaware of the fact that electroconvulsive therapy (ECT) is a safe and effective treatment for depression, especially for those depressions that are not responsive to antidepressant medicines. However, one of the side effects of ECT is temporary confusion and memory loss, so it has to be used with caution in patients who already have a cognitive impairment. Despite such possible side effects, research has shown that ECT can be an effective treatment for depression in dementia patients and can lead to improvements in both mood and cognition.

POTENTIAL BENEFITS AND RISKS OF SUPPLEMENTS

Linda felt that Ron's medicines were not improving his memory, so she turned to supplements as an alternative therapy. Approximately one out of every four people age 50 or older takes a supplement for brain health. Surveys also indicate that people who use dietary supplements tend to live healthier lifestyles by exercising, avoiding cigarettes, and eating nutritious diets. The AARP's Global Council on Brain Health recently reported that sales of supplements claiming to improve memory have almost doubled from 2006 to 2015. The annual sales of brain health supplements for 2016 totaled $3 billion.

A major problem with dietary supplements is that the level of scientific evidence supporting claims is much lower than for prescription medicines. Although regulatory guidelines vary in different parts of the world, in most countries it is possible to market dietary supplements and make claims about them without getting confirmation from double-blind placebo-controlled studies in humans. As a result, many consumers waste their money on products that may only be offering a temporary placebo effect.

Another issue with supplements is that people often assume that if a product is natural, then it is safe, but even natural dietary supplements can have side effects and interact with drugs in a way that decreases or increases the effects of those medications. For example, ginkgo biloba can interact with coffee to cause blood clots in the brain (i.e., subdural hematomas). It can also affect insulin secretion, making it risky for diabetics. Anyone interested in taking supplements for brain health should check with their doctor to ensure that they don't cause side effects or drug interactions.

Vitamins that are fat soluble, like A, D, E, and K, are not eliminated quickly from the body. Taking high doses of such fat-soluble vitamins should be avoided because it can lead to potentially harmful buildups in the body's fat tissue over time.

In 1994, the Dietary Supplement and Health Education Act set forth standards for manufacturers and distributors and prohibited them from marketing poor quality or misbranded products. Manufacturers are required to evaluate the safety and labeling of their products before they market them, but they are not required to perform double-blind, placebo-controlled studies in humans. Scientific evidence does suggest that some supplements might temporarily boost memory abilities in people with mild symptoms, yet many people still take them for more serious conditions like Alzheimer's dementia. However, because of the concerns about risks and limited evidence of memory benefits, some experts question whether these supplements should be taken at all.

Before taking a memory supplement, it's important to get accurate information about the brand reliability, effectiveness, and any potential side effects. I recommend talking with a knowledgeable pharmacist or physician. Information is also available from the National Center for Complementary and Alternative Medicine (nccam.nih.gov) and AARP's Global Council on Brain Health's recent report on brain health supplements (https://www.aarp.org/health/brain-health/global-council-on-brain-health/supplements/).

Many supplements that have been used to improve memory and bolster brain health are thought to exert their effects through various mechanisms, such as reducing oxidative stress or fighting inflammation. The following summarizes what is known about some of the more popular brain health supplements.

DID YOU KNOW?

Research has shown that people who take statins for high blood cholesterol levels do have a slower rate of cognitive decline as they age. However, on rare occasions, statins can cause memory side effects. One study of people who had cognitive side effects after starting statin therapy showed improvements in cognitive complaints after discontinuing their statin. Anyone thinking of discontinuing a medication because of possible side effects should first check with their doctor.

Anti-inflammatory Supplements

Inflammation is a natural physiological process that repairs tissue damage and helps fight off infections. As the brain ages, however, it experiences excess inflammation that contributes to dementia and cognitive losses, so the brain needs ways to fight back.

Many people take anti-inflammatory omega-3 supplements, which are made from fish oil, krill, or algae. People with higher blood levels of omega-3 fat have larger brains, especially in their hippocampal memory centers. Two essential omega-3 fatty acids, eicosapentaenoic acid (EPA) and docosahexaenoic acid (DHA), are necessary for normal brain development. Despite their anti-inflammatory effects, omega-3 supplements have not been shown to benefit patients who already have dementia.

In nondemented people, the scientific evidence suggests that dietary omega-3 fats fight brain inflammation and may boost memory as well as mood. People who consume omega-3 fatty acids have a lower risk of cognitive decline as they get older, but many of us do not get enough omega-3 fats from our diet.

Epidemiological studies have shown that consuming anti-inflammatory spices may protect brain health. In India, where they eat a lot of curry and other spices, the prevalence of Alzheimer's dementia in people in their 70s is four times lower than in the United States. Curcumin, a component of the spice turmeric and curried foods, has received recent attention as a brain health supplement in part because of its anti-inflammatory effects.

In addition to fighting inflammation, curcumin is an antioxidant and fights against the amyloid and tau proteins that build up in the brain and characterize Alzheimer's disease. Our UCLA research team recently studied a bioavailable form of curcumin (Theracurmin), which is well absorbed into the bloodstream. In our 18-month study of Theracurmin (using capsules that contain 90 milligrams of curcumin that are given twice daily), we found that nondemented middle-aged and older adults experienced better memory and attention than did control subjects taking a placebo. Even though this promising study was well-controlled, we are planning to replicate it in a larger group of volunteers to confirm our initial findings. In the meantime, many people concerned about brain health have begun consuming spicy foods or taking curcumin or turmeric supplements because of the potential benefits and minimal risks.

Antioxidants

As the brain ages, oxidative stress escalates and attacks neurons, causing wear and tear on these brain cells. Antioxidant vitamins have been used to reduce oxidative stress and protect brain health. Two decades ago, investigators reported that 2,000 units of the antioxidant vitamin E taken daily slowed the progression of Alzheimer's dementia in patients. As a result, doctors began prescribing these high doses of vitamin E to their patients with dementia, and many people with mild forgetfulness started taking high doses of vitamin E.

Later research, however, showed a link between taking more than 400 daily units of vitamin E and serious cardiac events, along with a greater risk of death. This 2005 report caused public concern, and the medical profession backed off from using high-dose vitamin E, especially in older individuals with a history of heart disease. However, a more recent study did support the brain benefits of vitamin E for mild to moderate Alzheimer's dementia, and the investigators did not observe cardiac side effects.

Even though taking vitamin E may benefit patients with mild to moderate Alzheimer's dementia, no study has ever shown that it has any effect on preventing Alzheimer's disease or delaying its onset in people with normal aging or mild memory symptoms. Another issue with vitamin E is that it can increase the risk for dangerous bleeding, especially when taken with anticoagulants like warfarin (Coumadin).

For thousands of years, Chinese medical practitioners have used leaves from the ginkgo biloba tree to treat heart and brain health problems. More recently, many people have taken ginkgo to improve their memory and mental focus. Studies show that ginkgo is an antioxidant that can increase brain circulation and enhance sugar absorption into brain cells. But ginkgo can cause side effects, including upset stomach, dizziness, headaches, bleeding, and lowering of blood pressure. Although earlier research demonstrated memory benefits for people with normal aging, a large six-year study failed to demonstrate any cognitive benefits in older, nondemented adults.

Several other antioxidant supplements have been used for boosting memory. Laboratory and animal studies suggest cognitive benefits from taking acetyl-l-carnitine and coenzyme Q10, but whether they actually boost brain health in humans is uncertain. Also, coenzyme Q10 increases the risk for blood clotting in people taking high blood pressure medications. Studies of vitamin C and beta-carotene have not shown consistent brain-protective results.

B Vitamins

The B vitamins include thiamin (B1), riboflavin (B2), niacin (B3), pantothenic acid (B5), pyridoxine (B6), biotin (B7), folate (B9), and cobalamin (B12). Because absorption of B vitamins can vary among individuals, these vitamins are generally included in multivitamin supplements.

Our brains need folate, or folic acid, for proper nerve function. Green leafy vegetables contain folate, and many breads and cereals are enriched with it because folic acid deficiency during pregnancy can lead to birth defects. Although folate may protect older adults from developing strokes and heart disease, folate supplements have not been shown to improve memory or prevent dementia. Also, too much folate may impair memory in older people who have low vitamin B12 blood levels.

Homocysteine is an amino acid building block of protein. When the body processes homocysteine, it produces vitamins B6, B12, and folate. High homocysteine levels in the blood are associated with a greater risk for developing Alzheimer's dementia. A two-year study from Oxford University showed that vitamin B supplementation in patients with mild cognitive impairment led to slower cognitive decline and slower shrinkage of the brain than use of a placebo.

About one in ten older adults may be deficient in vitamin B12, which can lead to depression, memory impairment, fatigue, and numbness and tingling in the hands and feet. If you have such symptoms, check with your doctor, who can draw blood levels and determine if B12 supplementation is indicated.

Vitamin D

Sunlight provides our bodies with vitamin D, but many people spend much of their time indoors and are deficient in this vitamin. Dietary sources of vitamin D include milk products and fatty fish like salmon and tuna, but not everyone consumes these foods. Vitamin D deficiency is an issue for some older individuals, and it is linked to cognitive decline. Your doctor can check to see if you have adequate vitamin D levels. A study of approximately 5,000 older women showed that those taking the recommended weekly amount of vitamin D had better cognitive function than those who did not. However, other studies have not replicated these results, so the evidence is limited for recommending vitamin D supplementation to boost brain health in people without a deficiency.

Melatonin

This hormone has been used to help people achieve restful sleep, and a good night's sleep is important for optimal cognitive functioning. Several studies have shown that melatonin can reduce the amount of time necessary for falling asleep as well as increase the total amount of sleep time and degree of sleep quality in people who have sleep disorders. It may also improve alertness in the morning. Although melatonin may offer benefits for sleep, whether it actually improves memory and brain health is uncertain.

SUPPLEMENTS USED FOR MEMORY AND BRAIN HEALTH

- *Anti-inflammatory supplements*. Omega-3 fatty acids (fish oil), curcumin
- *Antioxidants*. Vitamin E, acetyl-l-carnitine, coenzyme Q10, ginkgo biloba
- *B vitamins*. Folate (vitamin B9), cobalamin (vitamin B12)
- *Vitamin D*
- *Melatonin*
- *Phosphatidylserine*
- *Huperzine A*
- *Apoaequorin*

Phosphatidylserine

Phosphatidylserine is a chemical that is needed for normal cellular communication, and many studies suggest that it may benefit cognitive function. For example, a three-month study of older adults with mild memory symptoms showed that taking a phosphatidylserine supplement along with an omega-3 fatty acid benefitted memory abilities better than a placebo. Other studies have shown similar benefits without the additional omega-3 fatty acid supplementation. However, larger studies have not confirmed that phosphatidylserine supplements help prevent cognitive decline or improve memory.

Huperzine A

Extracts of firmoss plants contain Huperzine A and have long been used in China for treating swelling, fever, and blood disorders. Huperzine A may also boost brain levels of neurotransmitters, including the brain messenger acetylcholine, which is depleted in Alzheimer's disease. Earlier research has demonstrated its effectiveness in patients with dementia as well as milder cognitive problems, but other studies contradict those findings. The scientific evidence is inadequate to recommend using Huperzine A supplements for treating age-associated memory loss or dementia.

Apoaequorin

Most people have seen the television ads for Prevagen, which contains an ingredient originally derived from jellyfish and is thought to support brain health. The Apoaequorin protein isolated from the *Aequorea victoria* jellyfish has been studied in one clinical trial, which showed improved cognitive function in older individuals. However, that study had no placebo-control group. Another clinical trial did not demonstrate statistically significant improvement in the experimental group compared with a placebo group as a whole. Moreover, the chemical structure of the active ingredient of Apoaequorin is probably broken down in the gut before it reaches the brain. So despite the company's heavy advertising campaign, there is inadequate scientific evidence that it helps with memory and brain health.

CHAPTER 4

Practical Strategies for Caregivers

There are only four kinds of people in the world. Those who have been caregivers; those who are currently caregivers; those who will be caregivers; and those who will need a caregiver.

—Rosalyn Carter

MOST PEOPLE DO NOT relish the idea of having to accept care from others, even when that care is offered in a loving way. Receiving care translates into having to give up autonomy—an awful thought to most people, particularly those who are used to being in charge of their own lives. Many patients in the early stages of dementia lie about their symptoms in order to preserve their independence and avoid worrying their loved ones. However, when someone's diminishing mental capacity threatens their safety and that of others, a caregiver must intervene.

Caregiving for a patient with dementia is a daunting job. There's no formal course on how to do it, and it's impossible to anticipate the multitude of challenges you will face as the patient's dementia advances.

Keeping in mind a few practical strategies for dealing with some of the common issues that emerge in caregiving can make a huge difference in reducing the emotional burden and optimizing the patient's care. It can also benefit the well-being of both the patient and the caregiver.

DID YOU KNOW?

Dementia caregivers are at increased risk for cardiovascular diseases, especially hypertension, and approximately 40 percent of them have symptoms of depression and anxiety.

When trying to help a patient with dementia, it's important to remember that even the simplest tasks can trigger frustration—for both parties. Caregivers who can anticipate that small tasks take longer for patients with dementia will have an easier time completing those chores. Providing simple instructions and keeping daily activities as routine as possible can also reduce frustration. Offering patients some choices gives them a sense of empowerment that further facilitates caregiving, although too many choices can be confusing. When caregivers are flexible and resilient, patients often experience less stress and irritation.

TAKING AWAY THE CAR KEYS

During the course of my career as a geriatric psychiatrist, I've found that having to take car keys away from a patient who has become too cognitively impaired to get behind the wheel is perhaps one of the most challenging tasks. Most people, even those who are moderately demented, can usually recall their 16th birthday or whatever date they were allowed to start driving alone. This major coming-of-age milestone is symbolic of independence and autonomy. It follows, then, that relinquishing that privilege can be an anxiety-provoking and often dreaded event.

A few years ago, I got a frantic call from my cousin. Her 79-year-old mother had caused two fender benders in the last month, and that morning she hit three parked cars while driving out of a lot. Fortunately, no one was hurt, but my cousin's mother blamed the accident on a made-up mechanical problem that didn't actually happen. She insisted she wasn't at fault, but her car was in the body shop for the third time. I encouraged my cousin to keep her mother off the road until her driving skills could be properly assessed.

Driving allows older adults to remain mobile and independent, and losing the right to drive is a clear signal that the future holds only greater and greater reliance on others. Like my cousin's mother, many older drivers get defensive about their skills and are adamant about continuing to drive themselves at all costs, even when their cognitive skills are diminishing.

Although older drivers often have more experience and better judgment than many reckless teenage drivers, advancing age definitely impacts reaction time, visual acuity, and other mental skills, which can increase the risk for accidents. Laws about driving for people with cognitive impairment vary from state to state. In California, for example, physicians are required to report patients with cognitive impairments that may impair their driving to the Department of Motor Vehicles. Other states may not be as strict, but the California law is designed to protect the physician, patient, family, and public.

Research shows that elderly drivers with mild to moderate dementia have significantly greater risks for car accidents when compared to those not demented. A longitudinal study of drivers with dementia confirmed the decline of on-road driving abilities, especially those skills requiring more complex cognitive actions, such as awareness of driving environment and decision making.

SIGNS OF DRIVING TROUBLE

- ☐ Delayed reaction times
- ☐ Difficulties turning, especially left turns
- ☐ Driving too fast or too slow
- ☐ Hitting curbs
- ☐ Other drivers honking
- ☐ Problems changing lanes
- ☐ Multiple dents and scrapes on the car
- ☐ Trouble following signals and signs

Whenever I am concerned that a patient's cognitive abilities may be interfering with their driving, I inform the family that unless they ensure that the patient discontinues driving until properly assessed for driving skills, I am required by law to report them. It is often a sensitive topic, but I appeal to their sense of civic duty to protect themselves and the public. I remind them of another motivation for a proper assessment: it will protect their financial assets. If the cognitively-impaired driver did get into an accident, the family could be sued for damages and the patient's medical history would likely become a legal vulnerability.

TIPS FOR CONFISCATING THE CAR KEYS

- During the conversation, avoid saying "We think you should stop driving" and instead ask, "What do you think we should do?"

- Emphasize that you want them to continue living an active life

- Share your fears about them having an accident

- Involve a neutral third party, such as a therapist, family doctor, or aging specialist

- If possible, encourage them to try taxis, Uber, Lyft, or some other transportation alternative

- If necessary, get creative:
  - Hide the car keys
  - Disable the vehicle
  - Keep the car somewhere else
  - Sell the car

DEMENTIA AND RETIREMENT

The problems with concentration, mental flexibility, and abstract thinking that are characteristic of dementia impair a person's ability to carry out job duties. Because of the shame and embarrassment many patients feel, they often try to hide their difficulties from others while worrying about their financial future.

IF DEMENTIA INTERFERES WITH WORK

- Consult your doctor, who may identify a treatable cause for your symptoms or prescribe a medicine that may temporarily stabilize them so you can stay on the job longer.

- Your doctor may provide a certificate of incapacity to work so you can stop working without it affecting your pension.

- If it is safe and you can make adjustments to your job duties, try to continue working for as long as you can.

- Consider early retirement or a less-demanding position.

- Consider discussing your diagnosis with your union or employer.

- You may wish to share your challenges with work colleagues to help them understand your diagnosis and limitations.

For some patients, it is possible to cut back on their job tasks so they can remain active in the workforce longer, but eventually the patient will need to retire or resign. Also, losing driving privileges can interfere with people's work duties and often lead to job termination. The decision to leave the job is usually a huge emotional challenge for patients and their families. For many people, work means more than just earning money. It is a part of their identity and offers meaning and structure to their lives. After retirement, hobbies or volunteer work become critically important for anyone, with or without dementia.

MONEY MATTERS

As the patient's cognitive abilities continue to decline, at some point it will become challenging and eventually impossible for them to manage their finances on their own. For some patients, money problems can be one of the first indications of the disease. Paying bills and balancing checkbooks become difficult, and many patients attempt to hide their financial problems in order to protect their independence.

Early signs of financial struggles might include having trouble counting change or calculating a tip. Other clues may be unpaid and unopened bills lying around, odd credit card purchases, or money missing from a bank account. When money problems emerge, it is best to designate a family member or trustee to hold title to the patient's property and funds and check bank statements and other financial records at regular intervals.

Many older adults become victims of financial frauds involving identity theft, insurance scams, and get-rich-quick schemes. Anna, an 85-year-old grandmother with mild dementia, was still living on her own when she became a victim to such a scam. She called her daughter Donna to find out if her grandson Tyler had gotten back from his Mexico trip safely.

"Tyler didn't go to Mexico, Mom; he's here working all summer."

"But the American Embassy in Mexico called me. They said he'd been in a car accident and needed $1,400 to pay the fine and get his car back."

"That's impossible, Mom."

"But I talked to him myself, dear. The poor thing begged me not to tell you about it because he didn't want to get into trouble. So I wired him the money."

Anna had fallen victim to a common scam perpetrated on grandparents and other relatives. Usually someone pretending to be from a foreign embassy or police station calls to say that the grandchild is in some type of trouble and needs money quickly. The phony relative may actually get on the phone and feign being sick or upset to disguise their voice and sound convincing. Victims usually report that they were sure they were talking to the actual relative. This ruse has become so common that the US Department of State has a warning on its International Travel website about "grandparents scam" and how to avoid it.

After the scam incident, Donna became more insistent about her mother's immediate safety and care, and Anna was more realistic about accepting the help. When Anna heard about how many older people had been duped by this grandparent's phone scam, she didn't feel quite as foolish and ashamed of her error.

Donna found a service that provided supervision and care for her mother at home. She took Anna to a specialist who diagnosed mild Alzheimer's dementia and prescribed a memory medicine that did not upset her stomach. Anna's mind seemed a little sharper and everyone in the family noticed that Mom wasn't repeating herself as much. At least for now, while her memory was a bit better, Anna knew to be more cautious when someone wanted something from her, especially over the telephone.

HOME SAFETY STRATEGIES

The cognitive changes associated with dementia can create safety hazards in the home. Patients may forget to turn off an oven, stove, or portable space heater. They may wander off, get lost, and become victims of crime. As dementia progresses, gait instability is common and can lead to falls and injuries.

FALL PREVENTION TIPS

- *Bathroom safety.* Install grab bars in the shower and tub and place rubber mats in bathtubs and on shower floors.

- *Declutter.* Identify anything that could cause a trip or fall, such as small furniture, pet bowls, electrical cords, or throw rugs.

- *Create walking paths.* Rearrange the furniture so it's easy to navigate from one room to another.

- *Secure carpets.* Replace slippery area rugs with nonslip ones or use double-sided tape to attach the rugs to the floor.

- *Keep floors dry.* Use nonskid floor wax and search for any dripping faucets that could create puddles and tripping hazards.

- *Keep it light.* Visual acuity declines with age, so use high-wattage bulbs to ensure adequate lighting throughout the house to reduce the risk of falling.

- *Install handrails.* To help patients maintain balance and avoid falling, handrails are essential for stairs and other risky areas of the house.

- *Night safety.* Keep a flashlight and slippers at the bedside. Nightlights throughout the house will help patients avoid falls.

The first step in ensuring a patient's safety is to inspect and evaluate the home environment. Some areas may be particularly risky, such as garages, work rooms, basements or any area with chemicals, tools or other potentially harmful items.

Older patients with dementia are eight times as likely to fall compared to nondemented older adults. Getting rid of household hazards can prevent fires, slips, and other accidents that commonly occur at home.

You can install a hidden gas shut-off valve or circuit breaker for the stove and oven to prevent the patient from turning them on. Also, switch to appliances that have auto shut-off features. Keep medicines in locked cabinets and remove all firearms from the home.

When something is out of sight, it is also out of mind, so place deadbolts either high or low to make it harder for the patient to wander out of the house. Also get rid of or disable bathroom or bedroom locks so the patient doesn't get locked in. You can further ensure safety at home by checking with the doctor to make sure medications are not reducing the patient's sensory acuity or worsening confusion.

STRATEGIES FOR REDUCING AGITATION

As cognitive decline progresses in patients with dementia, they often develop agitation that can be difficult for caregivers to manage. Many patients experience restlessness and may start pacing. Others express their agitated feelings verbally by complaining or shouting. Sometimes agitated patients may escalate and become aggressive, which can pose a risk of injury for both patients and their caregivers.

Agitation may stem from anxiety or psychotic symptoms that are disturbing for patients and caregivers. The patient's healthcare provider should search for medical causes of agitation, such as infections, medication side effects, or metabolic disturbances. Treating such underlying conditions may reduce or even eliminate the symptoms.

The likelihood of agitated behavior increases following a move to a new residence or long-term care facility. In fact, any change in the patient's environment—travel, hospitalization, houseguests, or new caregivers—can lead to agitation.

Antipsychotics, antidepressants, anticonvulsants, and other medicines may help diminish these symptoms, but nonpharmacological approaches are preferred in order to avoid medication side effects. Caregivers can have an important impact on minimizing agitated behavior by practicing some practical techniques.

Should the patient become agitated, assess the immediate environment and eliminate any potential agitation triggers including noise, glare, extreme heat or cold, or a loud television. Also check for physical triggers like pain, constipation, a full bladder, or skin irritation.

Providing opportunities for physical exercise can help. Working in the garden, taking walks, and even dancing can provide a physical and emotional outlet that can help reduce agitated behaviors.

INTERVENTIONS FOR REDUCING AGITATION

Aromatherapy

Art therapy

Dancing

Exercise

Hearing aids

Light therapy

Massage

Music therapy (listening, singing)

Outdoor walks

Pet therapy

Reality orientation

Relaxation training

Reminiscence therapy

Social interaction

Tai chi

Wandering areas

Because a patient's agitation often makes their caregivers feel anxious, it's important for caregivers to recognize their own anxiety and rather than becoming agitated themselves, remain calm. Slowing things down, speaking in a soothing voice, and trying to distract the patient from their agitation trigger can be effective. It is important to avoid showing alarm, raising your voice, or arguing with the patient. A reminder of a pleasant memory or playing calming music can be effective as well.

PERSONAL HYGIENE

As dementia symptoms progress, patients typically forget about bathing, changing their clothes, and other aspects of personal hygiene. Providing bathing assistance can be particularly challenging because it is such a private activity. Some people feel embarrassed about undressing and bathing in front of others and refuse to bathe altogether to avoid embarrassment. Covering mirrors, closing curtains, and maintaining a sense of privacy are important strategies to reduce such feelings. Making sure the bathroom is warm and playing relaxing music can also help the patient feel more comfortable while bathing.

Whether it's bathing, brushing teeth, or getting dressed, breaking down the tasks into simple steps will make it less complicated for the patient. Also, try giving the patient choices by asking whether they prefer a bath or shower.

Other hygiene tasks that may require caregiver assistance include toileting, hair care, ear care, and nail cutting. For all of these activities, it's important to help the patient do as much for themselves as possible. Also, approaching the patient with sensitivity, reassurance, and patience can assist in overcoming the patient's discomfort and resistance.

GETTING HELP

Many caregivers find it difficult to ask others for help. They may be concerned that even close friends or family members will turn them down, or perhaps they don't want to bother others with their personal problems. However, going it alone as a caregiver can be stressful and grueling. People who have the courage to ask others for help are often pleasantly surprised by the willingness of friends and relatives to pitch in and lessen the caregiving burden.

Attending support groups with other dementia caregivers is critically important for providing emotional and practical support. The Alzheimer's Association (www.alz.org) organizes such support groups throughout the US. Caregivers who attend support groups report feeling less isolated. They often gain a sense of empowerment and a better understanding of what to expect in the future, and their caregiving skills actually improve.

As the caregiving burden escalates, however, it may be necessary to hire part-time or even full-time help. Several kinds of professionals are available to assist with a loved one's care.

OPTIONS FOR HIRED CAREGIVERS

- *Personal care assistants* are unlicensed and relatively inexpensive caregivers with varying levels of experience and training. They can serve as helpers, drivers, or companions.

- *Home health aides* can monitor vital signs and assist with light housekeeping, bathing, dressing, and using the bathroom.

- *Licensed nursing assistants* and *certified nursing assistants* can take vital signs, set up medical equipment, change dressings, clean catheters, and administer some treatments.

- *Skilled nursing providers* are state-licensed providers who can observe and evaluate the patient's care and administer intravenous drugs, tube feedings, and injections.

- *Registered nurses* have met the state's licensing requirements and can provide direct care.

To get started on hiring help, it's useful to consider the patient's personality, particular limitations, and level of help needed. Recommendations from the doctor or referrals from friends can also be helpful. If the patient is covered by insurance, you may need a doctor's summary indicating the need for in-home care.

Many people enlist the help of an agency or caregiver registry to find a caregiver. Agencies will require a fee but can be helpful when replacing a caregiver if the patient's needs escalate. Useful resources are available online, such as AARP's Caregiving Checklist for Choosing an Agency for In-Home Care (www .aarp.org). Prescreened caregivers have passed prior background checks, but you will still want to inquire about relevant experience. Check to see if there's an employment registry in your area that provides lists of available nurses and aides who you can call directly.

Of course, when planning to hire someone, it's important to ask the right questions, so plan and write out your questions in advance. Be sure to contact references yourself because someone may seem great during the interview, but their references might convey a different view of them.

HOME ALONE VS. SENIOR LIVING

When it began to dawn on Ruth that her father's mind was gradually slipping, she began to envision full-time care in his future. Most of the family discussions about the practical solutions to Dad's growing need for help ended with his favorite line: "You're not putting me in an old folk's home; you'll have to carry me out of this house in a box."

Ruth could understand her father's anxiety about moving from his family home of 50 years to unfamiliar surroundings where he'd have to get along with strangers. She, too, had some concerns about her father moving because she'd read that patients with dementia can suffer worsening cognitive function when adapting to an unfamiliar living setting. However, living alone was becoming dangerous for Dad, and it placed a burden on the rest of the family to constantly visit him in order to counter the social isolation and loneliness that can accelerate cognitive decline.

When a burst pipe flooded her father's home, Ruth had no choice but to move him into a senior living facility. Her father fought hard to stay put in the house, but in the end, he acquiesced because he really had no choice. Once they got there, Dad immediately started griping about his room, the noise, the food, and all the "geezers" sitting around all over the place. Ruth calmed him down by saying that he only had to stay there while the house got repaired, although she knew that wasn't quite true. She stayed with him that evening until he fell asleep and then tip-toed out.

When Ruth returned the next day, she found her father in the dining room with two other elderly men. They were engaged in a loud discussion about politics, and her dad looked more engaged than he'd been in some time. Much to Ruth's relief, her father adjusted quickly to the new setting, made some new friends, and seemed to thrive in the facility. The move also relieved Ruth about the dangers of her father living alone with his progressing cognitive decline.

Some adult children invite their parents to move in with them and make alterations to their homes to accommodate their parent's privacy and safety needs. Even though it can sometimes be easier and cheaper to care for your parents in your home, it can get complicated if personalities clash in close quarters. Also, not all aging parents want to live with their children. A Gallup research project on aging and quality of life showed that although more than 50 percent of adult children would be willing to have their parent move in with them, less than a third of the aging parents said they would even consider it.

Many older adults opt for a continuing care retirement community, which provides residents with several different options from independent living to assisted living to full-time nursing care, depending on their current needs. Many of these communities resemble college campuses with educational courses, concerts, movies, and more.

TECHNOLOGY TO THE RESCUE

Advances in technology offer many options for older adults to maintain their independence despite progressive cognitive decline. Taking advantage of recent developments like ride-sharing apps and grocery delivery services can diminish the feelings of dependence and isolation. Today's seniors, however, are not always savvy technology users. For them, it can be a struggle to learn how to use these technologies late in life when it is most challenging because of diminishing mental and physical abilities. Effective use of the technology, therefore, may require assistance from tech-savvy family members, friends, or caregivers.

The Pew Research Center reported that in 2017, more than two-thirds of people 65 or older had internet access in their homes. For older adults who do use the internet, 71 percent of them do so on a daily basis. These trends indicate that older adults are catching up with younger adults in adopting technology; however, only about half of today's seniors own and use a smartphone. That can make it difficult for them to take advantage of services like Uber and Lyft on their own.

Despite such challenges, many assistive technologies are available to promote the patient's independence and reduce caregiver stress. The following are some to consider.

- *Electrical appliance monitors.* These technologies, designed for caregivers who do not live with the patient, monitor home appliances to alert caregivers if they have been left on.
- *Tracking devices.* Using GPS technology, these devices can be worn around the neck or wrist to keep track of patients with dementia who tend to wander off.
- *Home monitors.* This technology turns lights on and off and can change thermostat levels. They can also send alerts to the caregiver's smartphone to help ensure patient safety.
- *In-home cameras.* This is yet another way to monitor patients from afar. They help oversee the patient's general safety and ensure that they are taking their medications as prescribed. They can alert caregivers if no movement is detected after a set amount of time.
- *Clocks for dementia patients.* Patients with dementia often lose their normal 24-hour body rhythms and end up sleeping all day and staying up all night. Clocks designed for cognitively impaired patients are easy to read and help orient patients to the time of day.

- *Communication devices.* Many patients with dementia find modern cell phones and even landlines challenging to operate. Telephones adapted for ease-of-use can be preprogrammed with frequently called numbers. Video chat services like FaceTime and Skype can help patients with dementia remain in touch with loved ones who are too distant for visits. Some preprogrammed phones have space for placing photos of the person the patient wishes to call.
- *Reminder messages.* Recorded on a home device, these messages can be preprogrammed to remind the patient to take medicines and get ready for appointments.
- *Medication dispensers.* These can be low-tech pillboxes that mark the days of the week or more elaborate dispensers that beep and open to remind patients to take their medicines.
- *Home care robots.* This technology can assist human caregivers with housework, remind patients to take their medicines, and alert doctors if assistance is needed. Currently, these devices are rarely used but may be adopted more in the future.
- *Hearing aids.* Many older patients don't like these devices because of vanity or difficulty in using them. However, making sure that patients can hear will improve their general safety, level of mental stimulation, and overall quality of life.

CHAPTER 5

The Emotional Roller Coaster of Caregiving

I've learned that people will forget what you said, people will forget what you did, but people will never forget how you made them feel.

—Maya Angelou

ALICE'S MOTHER ALWAYS HAD trouble expressing her anger directly, and she was often passive-aggressive. Alice remembered one night when she was a kid: her family was watching TV after dinner and her sister noticed Mom wasn't there. They called out for her and searched the house to no avail. Alice finally found her sitting in the car in the garage, pouting and tearful.

"What are you doing in here, Mom?"

"Oh, somebody noticed? I thought I was just the cook and maid around here."

Rather than simply asking her daughters to help in the kitchen, she cleaned it herself and spent an hour sulking in the garage. Years later, when her mother was suffering from dementia and her cognitive abilities declined, this passive-aggressive trait morphed into outright aggression. She would startle the family with angry outbursts—lashing out at waiters for not bringing the bread fast enough or accusing their long-time housekeeper of stealing her misplaced hairbrush.

Alice's mom's dementia was altering the function of her brain's frontal lobe—the area responsible for controlling impulses. Its gradual shrinkage made it difficult for her to control the angry feelings that emanated from her amygdala, deep within the brain under the temples. As a consequence, her mental filters were disappearing.

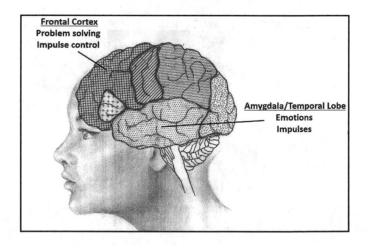

As Alice's mother's cognitive problems pro-gressed, she continued to deny what was going on and resisted her daughter's efforts to help. I see this in a lot of my patients, and it is always a struggle for their adult children who are caregivers. Occasion-ally though, an aging parent not only recognizes their deteriorating mental acuity; they are willing to accept assistance.

For example, my friend Stephanie's father, Errol, began developing Alzheimer's disease in his mid-70s. However, Errol was aware of his cognitive issues very early on and reached out to his daughter for help—even before Stephanie had acknowledged the problem. Stephanie remembered dropping by her dad's house on a Sunday afternoon. She had a key, so she let herself in.

"Dad? Are you home?"

"I'm back here in the bedroom, honey."

"Can I come in?"

"Okay, but it's a mess."

Stephanie walked down the hall to Errol's bedroom and found him sitting cross-legged on the king-sized bed surrounded by piles of papers, files, envelopes, receipts, handwritten spreadsheets, and canceled checks.

"What are you doing, Dad?"

"I'm was . . . I'm trying to . . ." Errol stared at the large envelope he was holding and seemed confused.

"Are you okay, Dad?"

"There's so many numbers." He started to tear up, and Stephanie went to hug him. She glanced at the papers and noticed several IRS 1099 forms.

"Are you doing your taxes?"

"Yes. That's right." Errol glanced around the room and asked, "What are all these papers for?"

"Don't worry, Dad," Stephanie said, "I'll help you sort it out."

COMING TO GRIPS: THE FIVE STAGES OF CAREGIVING

In her classic book *On Death and Dying*, Dr. Elisabeth Kübler-Ross described the five emotional stages that people typically experience when mourning the loss of a loved one. As our loved one's mental capacities begin to decline, we also begin to anticipate a loss—the loss of emotional support and unconditional love that we've known from them.

Most beginners on the journey of caregiving experience a range of unexpected and disruptive emotional responses that also emerge in five stages. At first these feelings can seem insurmountable and overwhelming, but almost all caregivers go through them. Those who are able to acknowledge their feelings and recognize that they are not alone will benefit by gaining perspective, insight, and confidence.

Denial

Denial is usually the first reaction to the idea that a loved one's memory issues are getting worse. In this stage, caregivers may think that they are imagining things, the diagnosis is a mistake, or somehow what they suspect is happening is really not.

To many, a loved one's initial forgetfulness seems normal at first, and they can handle that, but the idea of it getting much worse is unacceptable. Family members tend to play down the symptoms in the beginning—most are too busy with their own lives to make much out of a relative's repeated questions and social withdrawal. Ironically, when relatives do start to worry and encourage the patient to seek help, the patient's own denial—refusing to see a doctor, accusing relatives of conspiring against them, blaming others for their mistakes—further delays their getting help.

Denial is a psychological defense strategy that people use when reality becomes too painful to accept. Because memory defines who we are, it's no surprise that the threat of losing one's memory stirs up strong and primitive feelings that are intolerable on a psychological level. For adult children who become caregivers, the idea of losing their parental cheerleaders can be so painful that their minds deny it and refuse to accept the reversal of the traditional parenting roles.

To some extent, denial offers mental fortification. After all, if we constantly focused our attention on all the tragedy and pain in the world, it would be difficult to cope at all. But when it comes to a loved one's mental decline, we can only stay in denial for so long. Eventually it breaks down and the truth sets in.

An "aha" moment occurs when friends and relatives finally comprehend—intellectually and emotionally—what is happening to their loved one and what may lie ahead. Although the signs may be present long before the denial stage ends, there is usually a particular moment when caregivers suddenly grasp that their loved one's mental slips are no longer just "normal aging" but actual concerns to take seriously. Seeing the truth and fully accepting it, however, are two different things. Many people continue to struggle with their feelings and new responsibilities.

Emotional Turmoil

Getting a dose of reality about a loved one's mental decline often triggers intense emotions. Many caregivers feel depressed about the impending loss; some get angry that they now have to take care of their parent or spouse—it certainly wasn't a job they signed up for. That anger often stirs up feelings of guilt—"How can I be angry at my father? He's the one suffering from dementia!" Frustration is common because most people don't feel equipped to address the many medical, financial, housing, and other practical issues of caregiving. The stigma that still exists around dementia can also stir up feelings of shame and embarrassment.

Chasing a Cure

When our emotions get too intense, we often seek a quick fix to help manage them. Of course it's important to stay hopeful, but it's also essential to remain realistic about what can and cannot be done to help a family member with memory loss. Scientists are working hard to discover more effective treatments for encroaching dementia, but there is still no cure for the most common cause, Alzheimer's disease. Despite this fact, many adult children and spouses pursue exotic tonics and treatments to fix their loved one's brain. This pursuit of a magic bullet has taken families to Europe for stem cell cures or to Mexico for special potions that can only be found there. The flight to a fantasy cure can become very costly and can actually harm patients by delaying the use of conventional treatments that don't cure the disease but help stabilize symptoms.

Grief

When the aforementioned stages run their course and caregivers have accepted the reality of their loved one's mental decline, many begin grieving their loss. This can be a confusing stage—their loved one is present physically but becoming absent mentally. Patients in the late stages of dementia often experience sporadic moments of lucidity, which can complicate the grief process for many family members. It is not uncommon for adult children who are grieving to wish that their parent would finally die, and in fact, they may feel a sense of relief when their parent does pass away. Unfortunately that relief can sometimes be tainted by feelings of guilt about having wished for their parent's demise.

Acceptance and Resolve

The process of grieving helps family members come to grips with the truth of their impending loss. This usually allows them to pull it together and deal responsibly with the situation. Rather than riding an emotional roller coaster or pursuing groundless cures, they must acknowledge what they can and cannot do to help. Once acceptance and resolve set in, adult children and other caregivers are better able to make sensible and practical choices about caring for the patient. Arriving at this stage often frees up the caregiver's emotional energy so they can enjoy the time they have left with their loved one.

For most people, these five stages emerge in the order I've described. However, depending on the experiences, resources, and emotional strength of the caregiver, they may get stuck in or keep returning to one or more of the stages. It's also possible to skip one or two stages completely. Understanding that these stages are normal and giving yourself permission to experience and work through them is key to providing the best care possible for loved ones suffering from dementia.

CAREGIVING CAN BE DANGEROUS TO YOUR HEALTH

Whenever I consult with family members who are caring for their loved one with dementia, I am on the alert for signs of stress. Too many caregivers fail to take care of themselves, which can aggravate their own health and disrupt their caregiving efforts. Unbridled caregiver stress has many consequences, including sleep deprivation, poor eating habits, physical illnesses, and mood disorders. Family conflict and financial pressures add to this stress, and multiple studies have shown that the risk for significant depression in primary caregivers of dementia patients approaches 50 percent.

The stress of caring for a patient with dementia not only impairs the body's immune system; it also impacts telomere length, which is a biological marker of shortened life expectancy. The Alzheimer's Association and other organizations have highlighted some of the signs indicating that caregivers may be suffering from stress that threatens their physical and emotional health. These include getting angry at the patient; withdrawing from friends and activities that once brought pleasure; worrying about the future; experiencing physical health problems; and developing depression, exhaustion, insomnia, irritability, and impaired concentration. Any and all of these developments may indicate that it is time to consult with a mental health professional for help.

The greatest predictor of caregiver burden is the patient developing disruptive behaviors, such as agitation, aggression, and disinhibition. Despite the negative health consequences of stress, caregivers who learn to manage it effectively enjoy better moods, improved cognitive abilities, and even longer life expectancy.

TAKE A BREAK: RESPITE CARE

Taking regular breaks from any challenging task is essential for your emotional and physical health. Family caregivers can take those much-needed breaks by asking other relatives or friends to help out. They can also take advantage of respite care programs that provide primary caregivers with some temporary relief and can be arranged for one or more days a week, either in the home or at a facility.

A recent study evaluated the effectiveness of an in-home respite care program. Caregivers using in-home respite care were compared to control subjects who did not use respite care. After a six-month period, the respite care group had a significantly lower desire to institutionalize the patient compared with the control group caregivers as well as lower stress levels and a reduced burden on their social and family life.

Some caregivers express guilt about relying on respite care, but caregiving is demanding, and taking breaks allows caregivers to reduce their stress as well as their risk for depression. As a result, they can be more available emotionally to provide care while they are on duty. Respite care gives family members some time to relax, do their errands, and spend time with friends. It also can provide patients with opportunities to socialize and receive additional care from others.

Caregivers with limited resources may express concern about the costs of respite care services, but many programs offer scholarships and fees with sliding scales. A local Alzheimer's Association chapter can provide information on the availability of such financial assistance programs. Medicare and Medicaid may offer assistance as well. It's always a good idea to properly vet any program you are considering by ensuring that the staff are certified and well trained.

TYPES OF RESPITE CARE

- *Informal care at home* can be provided by friends, family members, or volunteers.

- *In-home care services* include companions, personal care assistance, homemakers, maid services, and skilled care to help with medication and other medical assistance.

- *Adult day centers* offer a safe environment for engaging in music, art, games, and other activities. Transportation and meals may also be provided.

- *Residential facilities* may offer overnight stays for patients.

GETTING REAL ABOUT CAREGIVER EXPECTATIONS

It is important for caregivers to manage their expectations. When caregivers remember that over time dementia patients will become more dependent and require higher levels of care, their expectations may be more realistic. When I meet with families, I try to help them plan for the future by educating and reminding them of some of the following realities of the disease:

☐ Alzheimer's disease has no cure.

☐ A reasonable goal is to temporarily stabilize symptoms.

☐ Despite stabilization, symptoms will eventually worsen.

☐ Be prepared for changes in symptoms and the emergence of new challenges.

☐ Caregiving is hard work, so make sure you take care of your own needs too.

☐ Anticipate the five stages of caregiving:
1. Denial
2. Emotional turmoil
3. Chasing a cure
4. Grief
5. Acceptance and resolve

☐ Expect that your loved one will change and that you will gradually mourn their loss as their dementia symptoms progress.

STAYING CONNECTED

Even though caregiving involves ongoing social contact between the patient and caregiver, the burden of the task takes up so much time and emotional energy that many caregivers feel isolated and alone. All humans, however, crave social contact, and staying connected to others is vital to maintaining mental health.

Remaining connected to friends and family members will reduce stress and lower the amount of cortisol and other stress hormones in your body. Chronic elevations of cortisol and other stress hormones heighten an individual's risk for age-related diseases such as Alzheimer's, heart disease, and diabetes—all conditions that threaten mental acuity. By contrast, social bonding and feelings of belonging increase the release of oxytocin, one of the brain's feel-good hormones.

Many studies have shown that spending quality time with family and friends actually extends life expectancy. For example, after following 3,000 older people for 10 years, researchers found that those who spent more time socializing had a 20 percent greater chance of longer survival than those who seldom or never socialized.

Maintaining close relationships with others makes us feel less alone and provides us with a sense of belonging. It can improve our mood and raise our self-esteem and confidence. Staying socially connected also exercises our brain cells. Having a conversation engages numerous neural circuits that control language and reasoning (located in the brain's frontal lobe) as well as emotions and memory (medial temporal lobe).

Remaining social may even slow age-related cognitive decline. Investigators have demonstrated connections between loneliness and dementia risk; however, becoming and staying socially engaged may reduce dementia risk by as much as 60 percent. Also, empathic responses during social interactions can lessen our worries and stress levels.

Caregivers who are feeling isolated and alone can improve their situation and caregiving effectiveness by paying attention to their friendships and close relationships. This will not only lower stress levels but also boost overall mental health. The following are a few strategies to consider:

- *Make time to talk.* Setting aside some time every day to talk to someone you are close to (perhaps scheduled as a regular time in the morning or evening) is an effective way to ensure that you maintain your emotional connections with those you care about. If you can't have an in-person get together, try video chatting or texting.
- *Lighten up with humor.* In most healthy relationships there will be arguments, but the key to successful relationships is *how* one argues. When you don't agree, try to punctuate your disputes with some humor and convey your understanding of the other person's point of view. Self-effacing humor is always safer than making fun of others.
- *Don't criticize.* The stress of caregiving can make people irritable and quick to criticize, but it's almost never welcomed. When you

focus on your friend's or partner's weaknesses, their first instinct will be to get defensive, which may sabotage your attempts to connect. If something in the relationship isn't working, try discussing the feelings that your partner's actions trigger in you instead of simply criticizing. Rather than saying, "Why do you slam doors while I'm working? You're so thoughtless," a better comment might be, "When I hear you slam the door, I feel distracted and annoyed."

- *Care for yourself.* Taking time to do things on your own will invigorate your sense of self and enrich your relationships. When possible, pursue your hobbies, go shopping, exercise, and take some time away from caregiving.

BEWARE OF DEPRESSION

Leonard, 74, closed the bedroom door after his wife Susan fell asleep. It had been a difficult evening. Susan refused to eat dinner and threw her plate at Leonard. He then had to change her soiled undergarments. When he tried to kiss her goodnight, she slapped his face.

Leonard sighed as he went to clean up the kitchen. Susan had been diagnosed with Alzheimer's disease six years earlier. At first she just repeated herself a lot and couldn't find the right words for what she wanted to say. But within two years she had lost most of her speech and became incontinent. Her gait became clumsy and soon she could only get around in a wheelchair.

Leonard was able to care for Susan on his own for the first three and a half years along with a little help from their daughter, Kara. And although they had labeled everything in the house and made other preparations, nothing could have prepared Leonard for the hell he was living now. He tried hiring aids and nurses to help out, but Susan hit them and yelled at them, and no one lasted very long. Susan rolled around the house in her wheelchair at all hours, moaning and wringing her hands anxiously.

Leonard was pretty sure Susan didn't know who he was anymore, and because he couldn't leave Susan alone in the house, he eventually stopped going out altogether. Leonard began experiencing headaches and fatigue, and sometimes he wept uncontrollably.

Kara was concerned that Leonard was depressed, and she feared for her father's health and well-being. She knew caregiving was stressful, but she had never seen Leonard so withdrawn, sad, and uncommunicative. It was time, she told him, to put Susan in a home where she could receive 24/7 care, and the stress of full-time caregiving would be off of Leonard.

Leonard initially resisted moving Susan, but Kara talked him into looking at some nursing homes in the area. They were lucky and found a facility with a great staff and a clean and homey environment. The residents seemed happy, and there were a lot of activities for them to engage in. The facility had a room available, but Leonard and Kara would have to act fast to secure it.

Leonard was ambivalent—he felt guilty about putting his wife into a home, but Kara said that his guilt was probably just a result of his depression, and she convinced him to move Susan to her new home. Leonard brought along Susan's favorite quilts, pictures, and other personal items to make her more comfortable. Susan moaned and resisted the help of the aids but eventually settled down and watched TV in the living room with the others. Leonard still felt horribly guilty about leaving Susan there, but in a few hours he went home and got the first full night's sleep he'd had in years.

Eventually, Leonard was able to get some professional help for his depression. Although he was ambivalent about it, moving Susan to a nursing home reduced his level of stress and improved his mood.

Leonard's experience with caregiving is common. A clinical depression requiring treatment from a health-care professional affects nearly half of all primary caregivers of patients with dementia. When caregivers accept help from others, take some time off for themselves, and set realistic goals, they are less likely to develop depression.

It's critically important to recognize depression because effective treatments are available. However, many caregivers do not seek help for their pain and suffering. Such depression can even put an individual's life at risk—patients whose depression is left untreated have a higher mortality rate from suicide or medical illnesses.

One reason that people fail to seek help is that depression distorts their thinking. When depressed, your mind plays tricks on you and impairs your insight, judgment, and reasoning.

When doctors assess a person for depression, they are looking for a cluster of symptoms that include the following: mood change (depression or anxiety or both), sleep disturbance (insomnia or increased sleep), loss of interest, feelings of guilt, low energy level, impaired concentration, appetite and body weight change (decreased or increased), agitation or slowed thinking and body movements, and suicidal thoughts. If a patient suffers from several of these symptoms, antidepressant medications, psychotherapy, or both can be very effective in relieving the symptoms.

The specific form of treatment will vary according to the type of depression and symptom cluster. For example, if a patient has particular difficulty sleeping at night, the doctor may prescribe a sedating antidepressant to help with insomnia. A novel approach to depression with insomnia involves the use of cognitive behavioral therapy for insomnia (CBTi), which teaches patients focused, behavioral methods to help them overcome their insomnia without medications. Initial studies suggest that CBTi not only improves sleep; it also lifts symptoms of depression.

STRATEGIES FOR BEATING DEPRESSION

- *Recognize the symptoms*. These symptoms can be both physical (insomnia, weight gain, agitation, fatigue) and psychological (guilt, sadness, loss of interest, poor concentration).

- *Don't self-treat*. Many people do not recognize that they need help, so they self-treat with alcohol and drugs or even TV binge-watching.

- *Get regular exercise*. Physical exercise should not be a substitute for proven medical treatments for depression, but numerous studies have demonstrated the mood-elevating effects of cardiovascular conditioning.

- *Stay socially connected*. Loners don't do well when it comes to mood. Strong social networks are associated with lower rates of depression.

- *Join a support group*. Caregiver support groups provide not only practical support but also emotional support, which will lower your risk for depression.

- *Get professional help*. Although depression is a treatable condition, at least half of those who experience symptoms do not get help. Remember that a variety of effective treatments and lifestyle strategies can improve symptoms.

CHAPTER 6

Lifestyle Habits That Protect Your Brain

---

*Whenever I feel like exercising, I lie
down until the feeling goes away.*
—Fred Dean, former NFL player

SEVERAL YEARS AGO, MARTIN, a 71-year-old executive,
asked me to create a personalized brain health
program for him in hopes of improving his worsening memory. Because of his hectic schedule, Martin
requested that I meet with him at his home near
the university. After entering his house, I could see
that he had a large staff taking care of the details
of his life. I waited in the library and he rushed in
15 minutes later, appearing harried and apologiz-
ing for a crisis at work and his driver getting stuck
in traffic.

After reviewing Martin's history and assess-
ing his cognitive abilities, I determined that he was

experiencing mild memory decline typical for his age and didn't appear to be suffering from anything more serious like dementia. He showed me the online brain game sites he visited daily and described the weight-training workout he was doing with his trainer. During our discussion, he was interrupted by three urgent phone calls, and I noticed his high level of stress.

I had several ideas to help Martin enhance his healthy lifestyle and ramp up his memory training. I spoke with his personal assistant regarding Martin's frenetic schedule and his chef about his diet. Martin and I then reconvened in the library, and I laid out my plan.

Although Martin already did weight-training three times a week, he still needed to get some aerobic conditioning. I told him that simply walking 20 minutes each day—either outside or on a treadmill—would suffice. The studies showing a link between cardiovascular conditioning and brain health indicate that 90 minutes of brisk walking each week is associated with a lower risk for dementia.

I also suggested that Martin cut back on the time he spent playing online word games and focus more on learning practical memory methods to improve his everyday issues: remembering names and faces, recalling appointments, and remembering where he put things. I demonstrated some basic techniques that help people focus their attention, create mental images of what they want to recall, and associate those images with something meaningful so they become memorable.

Martin already ate a fairly healthy diet, but he needed to increase his antioxidant foods such as green leafy vegetables, fresh berries, and green tea and cut back on potentially harmful fats from butter and red meat. All of these suggestions seemed easy to Martin, and he readily agreed.

Martin was surprised when I told him that his high stress levels were probably contributing to his memory complaints. When people are stressed, certain hormones are released in the brain, making it harder to concentrate on new information and recall it later. We discussed a few stress-reduction techniques, including relaxation exercises, meditation, and yoga. I showed Martin a simple breathing exercise that he could do throughout the day by closing his eyes, breathing slowly, and focusing on his breath coming in and out for just a few minutes. Martin noticed immediate benefits—he felt calmer and more focused.

Over the next month, Martin's memory symptoms began to improve, but I noted that he remained fairly isolated in his personal life. A widower for almost 20 years, Martin rarely socialized with people outside of work, and he had lost touch with most of the friends he used to see when he was married.

Remaining emotionally connected with family and friends is a crucial component of a healthy brain lifestyle. Support and empathy from loved ones decrease our stress levels. Engaging in lively conversation is a form of brain exercise that helps keep our memory function intact, and when we spend time with health-conscious people, those tendencies rub off and we take on their healthy habits for ourselves. When Martin began socializing more, his symptoms continued to improve, and he soon had far fewer memory complaints than before.

Martin's personalized brain fitness program was a success thanks to his willingness to make some changes in his everyday lifestyle habits. Over time, he continued to enjoy playing online brain games, but by optimizing other behaviors—physical exercise, stress management, and social engagement—he improved his memory ability and likely lowered his risk for future cognitive decline.

At this time, the multiple scientific studies searching for an Alzheimer's dementia cure have not yet been successful. However, the results of research on the effectiveness of a healthy lifestyle to protect brain health and delay the onset of dementia are very compelling. Regular physical exercise, mental stimulation, balanced diet, and stress management are key strategies that not only slow age-related cognitive decline; they can actually improve mental function in many people. In fact, research shows that a healthy brain lifestyle can protect cognitive abilities even in those with more advanced challenges.

Our team at UCLA has developed a memory lifestyle program that helps people like Martin create brain-healthy habits that that are personalized for them and tailored to their individual needs and cognitive challenges. Most of these programs focus on people with mild, age-related memory complaints who are concerned that their cognitive issues will progress to something more serious.

The key to making lifestyle strategies work is to customize the program so it makes sense for the individual's level of cognitive decline. If a memory training exercise is too difficult for someone experiencing mild dementia, it should be made less challenging by adjusting it to that person's particular level of cognitive ability. This way, individuals will avoid becoming frustrated and giving up. On the other hand, for people with very minimal complaints, exercises that are too easy will be boring and quickly abandoned.

HELPING PEOPLE CHANGE THEIR HABITS

After many years of practicing psychiatry, I've come to appreciate how difficult it is for people to change. One of the most important determinants of success is the individual's motivation level. And, regardless of how much someone is motivated, having others around who are encouraging and supportive of healthy habits can be critical to success.

People who are noticing their declining memory abilities and are concerned about future cognitive decline are usually quite motivated. This is especially true if they have a close family member who has suffered from Alzheimer's disease or another form of dementia.

When families consult with me, usually one relative with impaired cognitive abilities is identified as the designated patient. However, other family members often have memory complaints as well, and all of them are likely to benefit from a brain-healthy lifestyle. I try to engage friends and relatives of the patient to adopt a brain-healthy lifestyle together. This strategy also reduces the stigma experienced by the designated patient.

It is never too late or too early to start protecting brain health, and the sooner people get started, the more they will benefit from their improved brain fitness. Even when we do find a cure for Alzheimer's, it will always be easier to protect a healthy brain than to repair neural damage once it is extensive.

Many people assume that exercise, nutrition, and other healthy lifestyle habits are only effective for people with very mild symptoms, but research shows that they can help patients with actual dementia. For example, multiple studies have shown that regular physical exercise not only improves levels of physical fitness and function but also boosts cognitive abilities in patients who are already suffering from dementia.

When families engage in healthy lifestyle habits together, they are able to support each other in altering their behaviors. Eventually those healthy behaviors will transition into habits that will protect brain health for the long haul.

THE BRAIN-HEALTHY LIFESTYLE

Previous research has focused on the impact of various modifiable risk factors on future cognitive decline. Investigators at the University of California, San Francisco, studied the impact of several of these modifiable factors and their potential to delay or prevent Alzheimer's dementia. A risk factor is something that increases one's chance of getting a disease, and some are considered modifiable risk factors because we can do something about them. The researchers calculated the effects on the rates of dementia by reducing the following modifiable risk factors: diabetes, hypertension, obesity, smoking, depression, low education, and physical inactivity. The researchers concluded that a 10 to 25 percent improvement in all seven risk factors could potentially prevent or delay from one to three million cases of Alzheimer's disease worldwide.

Our UCLA research group found that these modifiable risk factors also influence mild subjective memory complaints that often precede the onset of Alzheimer's dementia. Our group collaborated with Gallup-Healthways, which surveyed more than 18,000 people from across the US. We found that modifiable risk factors for Alzheimer's disease were also associated with memory complaints in young, middle-aged, and older adults. And as memory problems increased, so did the number of risk factors. This investigation and other studies suggest an additive effect for engaging in more than one healthy behavior. For example, we found that people who did not smoke reported fewer memory problems than those who did. People who reported engaging in regular exercise as well as not smoking were even less likely to experience memory problems.

Such research led scientists in Finland to perform a large-scale study to test whether changing lifestyle and behavior can have a future impact on brain health. The investigators set out to determine if enrolling older volunteers in a program of regular mental and physical exercise, healthy nutrition, and other brain-healthy activities would delay future cognitive decline.

The investigation, known as the Finnish Geriatric Intervention Study to Prevent Cognitive Impairment and Disability, involved randomly assigning more than 2,600 people (ages 60 to 77) at risk for dementia (e.g., high blood pressure or cholesterol, mild memory impairment) to either an intensive healthy lifestyle program (regular nutritional counseling, personalized diets, exercise programs guided by physical therapists, and cognitive training) or a control condition of regular health advice. After two years, the volunteers who received the healthy lifestyle intervention demonstrated significantly better cognitive abilities compared with the control group who only got health advice.

UCLA's Longevity Center has created several programs to help people engage in a healthy lifestyle to improve their memory performance and lower their future risk of dementia (www.longevity.ucla.edu). Some of these programs involve attending classes, while other programs are individualized to meet the personal needs of the participant. Each of these programs involves some of the most important strategies for protecting brain health, including physical exercise, mental stimulation, balanced nutrition, and stress management.

PHYSICAL EXERCISE

You don't have to become a triathlete to protect your brain from Alzheimer's dementia. One study showed that just 20 minutes of daily brisk walking will lower your risk. Exercise lifts mood because it boosts endorphins. Workouts also produce brain-derived neurotropic factor (BDNF), a protein that gets your brain cells to sprout new branches and communicate more effectively.

Research at the University of Illinois has shown that physical exercise will make your brain bigger, and a bigger brain is a better brain. Regular brisk walking not only improves attention and thinking; it also increases brain size and function. After six months of regular cardiovascular conditioning, middle-aged and older volunteers were found to have larger hippocampal memory centers compared to a control group that only did stretching without walking. Hippocampal size increased even more for volunteers who continued their walking routine for an entire year.

Other research has demonstrated that strength training provides additional cognitive benefits beyond aerobic exercise. I recommend making daily walks a habit. If you like sports, get into a routine of playing tennis or racquetball with friends. Join a gym or buy some exercise bands so you can also increase your muscle tone and strength. As we age, balance training becomes increasingly important to help us prevent falls and injuries.

Physical exercise routines, of course, need to be adjusted depending on the person's baseline strength and stamina levels. If you are a caregiver and want to work out with your loved one who has dementia, keep in mind that gait instability and physical frailty are common in older patients with dementia. It is often necessary to work with an experienced trainer or physical therapist to make sure that the patient's exercise routine is safe yet still challenging enough to provide a physical and mental benefit.

MENTAL STIMULATION

We can stimulate our minds by playing games, socializing, traveling, and engaging in other activities that give our brain cells a workout. Multiple studies have shown that greater educational achievement, speaking more than one language, or playing games like crosswords or Sudoku are associated with a lower risk for dementia. Whether you attended college or not, lifelong learning can also lower your risk for cognitive decline, and brain scan studies have shown that just a few weeks of cognitive exercise will strengthen neural circuits.

The best strategy is to find stimulating activities that you enjoy and to train but not strain your brain. If learning a language is too challenging, try chess or cards or board games. Also, when engaging in mentally stimulating activities with someone who has dementia, try doing mental tasks that are fun but not overly challenging.

EXERCISE YOUR NEURAL CIRCUITS

Try this brain teaser to stimulate your mind. Spell three words that allow you to go from the word DINER to MENUS by changing only one letter at a time, while also forming a proper word at each step:

DINER

_____

_____

_____

MENUS

See answer at end of chapter 6.

Computer Brain Training

People often ask about whether today's new technology worsens or improves brain function. The answer is that our devices do both. When they distract us, they interfere with memory, but some apps and games actually improve cognition abilities.

Our UCLA research team did a study on what happens in our brains when we search online for the very first time. To perform this study, we recruited older volunteers who had never done an internet search as well as an older control group with prior internet search experience. We then tracked their online brain activity with an MRI brain scanner.

When the internet-naïve volunteers searched online for the first time, we observed minimal brain activity compared with the extensive neural activity we saw when the internet-savvy people searched online. We believe that when people first search online or engage in any new mental task, they're not sure exactly what to do, so we see minimal activity. Once they have a little experience and figure out a mental strategy for the task, we see an upsurge in neural firing. Therefore, simply searching online can be a form of brain exercise.

Other studies have shown that computer apps and videogames can train our brains and improve our problem-solving skills, attention, and reaction time. In fact, games that train working memory may actually make you smarter. Working memory, a form of short-term memory, is what temporarily holds information in the mind long enough to use it, such as hearing a phone number and then dialing it right away. The research indicates that when you train your working memory, it can translate into an improvement in fluid intelligence—the capacity to think logically and solve problems. Other research shows that some computer games can actually improve multitasking skills.

Neuroscientists at the University of California, San Francisco, studied the game *NeuroRacer*, which involves steering an animated race car along a winding road while informative and distracting street signs pop up. The investigators found that older adults who played the game for four weeks improved their multitasking skills to the point where they performed at the same level as untrained 20-year-olds.

Also, surgeons who play video games make fewer errors in the operating room. It is likely that action games that train attention and reaction time also improve surgical skills, so even playing some videogames can be mental exercise that provides practical benefits.

MENTAL BENEFITS OF TECHNOLOGY USE

☐ Improved memory from games that train cognition

☐ Memory augmentation from retrieval of stored data

☐ Better multitasking skills

☐ Increased problem-solving abilities

☐ Faster reaction time

Although overuse of computers and smartphones can distract us and impair our memory, there are many helpful computer programs that augment our biological memory. They allow us to pick and choose the information we need to remember and what information we can store on our gadgets. Learning and practicing memory methods to better recall names and faces will help improve your social skills, but things like appointments, dates, birthdays, and other detailed information can be stored and rapidly retrieved by using electronic devices.

Techniques for Improving Memory

We can train our brains using memory methods that compensate for everyday forgetfulness. Most memory techniques involve three important tasks: focusing attention, visualizing the information we wish to remember later, and creating mental associations that link these visual images, making them easier to recall.

The biggest reason people don't remember things is that they are simply not paying attention, so exercises that help focus attention will immediately strengthen memory abilities. Creating mental images leverages the brain's innate visual skills, and our associations give the information meaning. If something is meaningful, it will be memorable.

These methods are useful for everyday memory tasks, like recalling where you parked your car. When I park in lot 3B, I may visualize three large bees hovering over my car. It's important to use visualizations that have personal meaning. I have an aversion to bees, so that image makes it easy to remember for me. However, if I park one level below in lot 2B, I might imagine William Shakespeare standing on my car reciting "to be or not to be."

The methods are also powerful in helping people remember names and faces. For example, if you meet Sue Bangel and she has bangs, that image can help you remember her last name. If she happens to tell you she's an attorney, her first name will be easy to remember as well, especially if she is a litigation attorney and can *sue* you.

MEMORIZE A TO-DO LIST

Try thinking up a story that links together all the items you want to memorize. For example, I had two errands: buy eggs at the market and pick up my pants at the dry cleaners. I was too busy to write them down, so I pictured myself carrying an egg that breaks in my hand and stains my slacks–sending them to the cleaners. Now, try to create your own story for remembering the following errands:

1. Pet store–buy dog food

2. Bakery–pick up a pie

3. Dry cleaner–drop off jacket

   To remember these four errands, the story I created went like this:

   While walking my dog to the *pet store* to buy dog food, I got hungry and stopped at a *bakery* for some pie. My dog leapt for the pie, causing it to go all over my jacket, which then had to go to the *dry cleaner*.

Staying Socially Connected

Remaining socially engaged with others is associated with better cognitive abilities as we age. Researchers at the University of Michigan studied cognitive abilities as a result of a stimulating discussion and found that compared to watching a sit-com rerun, a 10-minute conversation results in significantly greater improvement in memory and speed of mental processing.

Conversations are like mental calisthenics that bolster neuronal networks. By engaging in daily discussions on topics of interest, you keep your neural circuits agile. Consider adding a social element to other brain-healthy strategies, such as walking with a friend—it will get your heart pumping oxygen and nutrients to your neurons and your brain cells will get stimulation from the conversation. Also, discussing stressful issues with an empathic friend will further bolster your brain health. Loved ones with dementia maintain better cognitive skills when they spend time with friends and family, which is one reason to consider a senior living option for older widows and widowers who still live at home alone.

BALANCED NUTRITION

A healthy diet can help keep muscles strong and protect us from obesity and diseases like high blood pressure, heart disease, and diabetes. Even though the benefits of good nutrition are now common knowledge, many people continue to eat in a way that endangers their bodies and minds. Nearly half the population is overweight or obese, conditions associated with several physical illnesses that can threaten brain health.

Central obesity, or the fat cells around the waist that many people acquire as they age, promotes a heightened inflammatory reaction in the brain that appears to attack brain cells. When scientists examine the abnormal amyloid plaques found in Alzheimer's brains, they see evidence of inflammation.

Portion control helps us avoid obesity, which impairs cognition and shortens life expectancy. When obese people lose weight, they experience significant improvements in memory, which can often last for years.

People who go on extended fasts or fad diets that severely restrict calorie intake often deprive themselves of necessary vitamins, minerals, fibers, and other nutrients that their bodies need to function normally. By contrast, large-scale epidemiological studies have documented the brain-protective benefits of a Mediterranean-style diet that includes lean proteins like fish and chicken, fresh fruit and vegetables, and whole grain carbohydrates. Researchers at Columbia University found that volunteers who consumed a Mediterranean-style diet had a lower risk for developing mild cognitive impairment or dementia later in life. Scientists at the University of Miami performed MRI brain scans on volunteers and found that those who ate a typical North American diet (e.g., high in fats, processed foods) had more damage to small blood vessels in the brain that service white matter, which transmits signals between neurons. Those who adhered to a Mediterranean-style diet showed less injury to those important blood vessels.

I recommend a nutritious diet that includes reasonable portion control. Eating several small meals throughout the day (breakfast, lunch, and dinner, plus mid-morning and mid-afternoon snacks), helps people avoid that feeling of hunger that sets in when they go too long without food. It's also a good idea to combine healthy carbohydrates and proteins at every meal and snack. The carbohydrates will provide immediate energy while the proteins provide a sustained sense of satiety.

Omega-3 fats from fish and nuts fight brain inflammation. Fruits and vegetables combat age-related oxidative stress that causes wear and tear on the brain's neurons. Also, we need to avoid or at least minimize all those tempting chips, donuts, and cookies. These refined sugars and processed foods increase our risk for diabetes, which in turn doubles our risk for getting Alzheimer's disease.

---

10 NUTRITION TIPS TO KEEP YOUR MIND SHARP

1. *Set realistic goals.* If you make your diet too restrictive, it will be hard to stick to. Avoid fad diets and set reasonable goals so you can maintain your diet.

2. *Control portions.* Obesity puts you at risk for diabetes, Alzheimer's, and other illnesses that threaten brain health, so limit your caloric intake.

3. *Eat frequent small meals.* Rather than fasting all day and splurging at dinner, eat smaller portions at breakfast, lunch, dinner, and two between-meal snacks.

4. *Combine proteins and carbs.* At each meal or snack, combine healthy proteins and carbohydrates for an energy boost (carbs) and sustained satiety (proteins).

5. *Eat fruits and vegetables.* Eating five servings of fruits and vegetables each day will protect your brain cells from the wear and tear of oxidative stress.

6. *Consume omega-3 fatty acids.* These healthy fats protect your brain from inflammation. Fish, nuts, or flaxseed are excellent sources.

7. *Limit refined sugar and processed foods.* Minimizing these foods will lower your risk for obesity, diabetes, and other illnesses that can damage your brain.

8. *Moderate caffeine use.* Moderate use of coffee and tea is associated with a lower risk for Alzheimer's disease and other forms of dementia.

9. *Spice it up.* Flavor your food with herbs and spices for added antioxidant power to protect your brain and allow you to use less salt. Lowering salt intake will help you avoid brain-damaging high blood pressure.

10. *Know your triggers.* Certain foods trigger some people to overeat. Whether it's chocolate, ice cream, or bread, know your triggers and avoid them.

At UCLA, we studied the memory effects of pomegranate juice, which is a potent polyphenol antioxidant. Our double-blind, placebo-controlled studies suggest that nondemented middle-aged and older adults who drink eight ounces of pomegranate juice each day can experience changes in brain neural circuitry and memory improvement after one month. Our follow-up study showed benefits in visual memory after one year of daily pomegranate juice consumption.

There's other good news on the nutrition front. Alcohol in moderation is associated with better brain health. It may be that a glass of wine at dinner lowers stress, which protects our brains, or perhaps it's an ingredient in the alcohol that is beneficial.

Our research team found that a bioavailable form of the spice curcumin (from turmeric) staves off memory loss. Curcumin fights inflammation, and people who live in India (where they eat lots of curcumin) have a lower risk for memory decline. Whether you take a curcumin supplement or not, consider using turmeric and other spices to flavor your food. Epidemiological research has shown that people who eat spicy Indian food on a regular basis perform better on memory tests.

STRESS MANAGEMENT

Caregiving or any other form of stress has negative effects on mental health. Studies of small animals under chronic stress show that their brains' hippocampal memory centers shrink because of it. The animals also develop memory impairment.

---

10 TIPS FOR REDUCING CAREGIVER STRESS

1. *Ask for Help.* Many caregivers feel they need to do everything themselves, but going it alone definitely increases stress levels.

2. *Stay close to friends.* Maintaining your own personal relationships will help protect you against the potential isolation of caregiving.

3. *Schedule fun time.* Allow yourself to take breaks to read, work in the garden, watch television, walk the dog, or do any activity that is fun and relaxing.

4. *Join a support group.* Talking about your feelings and receiving practical advice from others with experience can provide emotional relief.

5. *Meditate.* Meditation lowers stress levels and improves mood while strengthening neural circuits and increasing mental focus.

6. *Try other relaxation methods.* Yoga, tai chi, deep breathing, and other techniques can also help people learn to relax and unwind.

7. *Get physical.* The endorphin boosts and anti-inflammatory effects of aerobic conditioning can rapidly reduce stress and improve your mood.

8. *Sleep well.* A good night's sleep optimizes brain health, improves mental clarity, and reduces stress.

9. *Get organized.* Simply reviewing your calendar and to-do list each morning can have a major impact on lowering stress and doesn't take much time.

10. *Remember to laugh.* Humor releases tension, quickly improves mood, and may even offer new insights and perspectives on caregiving challenges.

Human volunteers injected with the stress hormone cortisol experience temporary memory impairment. Many can't remember details of what they have just read. But the good news is that these kinds of stress-induced memory difficulties resolve when cortisol levels diminish.

Stress is also closely linked to depression, anxiety, and other mood changes. When people feel helpless due to the chronic stress of caregiving, they may give in to those feelings and turn inward, which further exacerbates their sadness. Caregivers can also become overwhelmed from the lack of outside support, and social isolation increases their risk for depression.

The good news is that meditation, yoga, tai chi, and other relaxation methods can reverse stress and improve mood and memory. Meditation actually rewires the brain and improves measures of telomere length on our chromosomes, which predicts longer life expectancy. Keep in mind that spending time with friends and getting a good night's sleep are other important strategies for reducing stress.

Whether you are a caregiver now or anticipate being one in the future, don't let yourself become a victim of stress. Many of these stress management strategies can be done with dementia patients, which can help your relationship move beyond just a caregiving interaction and also help protect your loved one's brain health. For example, a variety of meditation apps (e.g., Calm, Insight Timer) can be downloaded to a smartphone. Try setting aside a particular time each day to meditate with your loved one: you will feel closer and more relaxed as a result. Studies of meditation have shown that as little as 10 minutes each day can lead to functional brain changes that improve mood and memory.

TRY THIS STRESS-REDUCING MEDITATION

- Get comfortable in a chair and place your feet flat on the floor.

- Resting your hands on your thighs, let yourself settle and close your eyes.

- Take several deep, slow breaths in through your nose and then exhale out through your mouth.

- Concentrate on your breathing and notice how the air feels cool as you breathe it in and warm as you exhale.

- Feel your body relax as your mind grows peaceful.

- Continue the exercise for five minutes and keep focusing on your breathing.

- If your mind wanders, gently bring your attention back to your breathing.

- After five minutes, open your eyes and notice if you feel more relaxed.

Answer to brain teaser on page 138:

DINER

MINER

MINES

MINUS

MENUS

CHAPTER 7

New Research: Hope vs. Hype

It is easy to get a thousand prescriptions but hard to get one single remedy.

—Chinese proverb

WHEN MY PATIENT DENNIS first came to see me, he had just turned 70 and was very concerned about his memory. He was having trouble coming up with people's names, and he couldn't remember phone numbers and addresses that he used to know. It reminded him of his uncle's early signs of Alzheimer's disease, and Dennis was convinced he was getting it too. He had heard there were new drugs that could stop the disease, and he wanted to start taking them immediately.

After getting a thorough history, I told Dennis that before we could formulate a treatment plan, I wanted him to take a full battery of tests, including a blood workup, neuropsychological testing, and brain scan. Dennis reluctantly agreed, but I could tell he was disappointed that I didn't have some kind of magic pill he could take to fix him that day.

A week after taking the tests, Dennis came back to hear his results. Unfortunately, I had to report that he did indeed have mild Alzheimer's disease. After calming Dennis down, I explained that because his case was extremely mild, he could definitely benefit from making some basic lifestyle changes. I emphasized the importance of daily exercise, a Mediterranean-style diet, stress reduction, and other strategies. I also wanted him to start taking Aricept, a drug that would stabilize his symptoms and might even temporarily improve them.

Dennis said he would try all those things, but he wanted more. He asked if there were any new drugs in the works and to try any type of experimental treatment. I offered to look for a clinical trial he could enroll in, and we scheduled another appointment in a week.

Dennis canceled his next appointment, and I didn't hear from him again for six months. When he came back in, he appeared tired and had lost weight. Dennis said he'd been in Germany getting stem cell injections that were supposed to cure his Alzheimer's disease, but they didn't work, and now his memory was getting worse every day. He apologized for not following up on my suggestions and wanted to get started right away.

This time Dennis followed my recommendations, and the lifestyle changes along with the medication did improve his symptoms slightly. He particularly liked taking walks every morning with his wife and found that working with a memory coach helped him compensate for some of his short-term memory difficulties. Eventually, Dennis enrolled in a clinical trial of an experimental Alzheimer's drug treatment, which allowed him to continue following my recommendations during the trial.

Unfortunately, Dennis's foray to Europe for an unproven remedy had postponed his starting an effective treatment plan for six months while his symptoms progressed. This is an important reason why patients should avoid unverified cures and therapies that have not been tested against a placebo in well-designed studies. Research indicates that in general, the sooner a patient gets started on proven and effective treatments, the better that patient's outcome. In addition to losing precious time when effective treatments could have been helping, these unproven "miracle cures" can also do harm and cause side effects. The weight loss and fatigue that Dennis experienced could have been from the stem cell treatment he'd tried or possibly some other remedy he was taking that he had not disclosed.

SEARCHING FOR TREATMENTS
THAT MODIFY THE DISEASE

Volunteering for clinical research is critically important in helping find new and effective treatments
for Alzheimer's and many other mental health diseases. The good news is that many treatment trials
allow patients to continue with their approved anti-
Alzheimer's medicines that are considered the current standard of care. These new studies are searching
for interventions that provide benefits above and
beyond what we have today, and patients don't have
to lose time off of their already proven treatments
that help them maintain a higher level of functioning
for longer periods.

A recent review of Alzheimer's disease research
indicated a total of 132 experimental treatments in
clinical trials, which means that they are being tested
in human volunteers using established scientific
methods. Many of the medicines in these studies
target cognitive abilities, while others aim to treat
the psychiatric and behavioral symptoms associated
with the disease.

Nearly 100 of these novel treatments are being
tested to determine if they are *disease-modifying*,
which means that they affect the underlying causes
of the disease and offer a benefit on the disease
course. Approximately 40 percent of these experimental treatments are designed to eliminate the

abnormal amyloid protein deposits that accumulate in the brains of Alzheimer's patients. About 20 percent of the treatments are targeting the abnormal tau proteins. Some of these various treatments are pills, while others are antibodies that are delivered intravenously.

VOLUNTEERING FOR A CLINICAL TRIAL

Unfortunately, the vast majority of Alzheimer's disease interventions tested thus far have failed. As a result, several major pharmaceutical companies have abandoned their search for new treatments for the disease. However, there are still many companies, research institutes, and academic centers that are vigorously pursuing innovative ways to tackle this devastating disease.

The only successful treatments thus far are categorized as symptomatic drugs, including Aricept (donepezil), Exelon (rivastigmine), and Namenda (memantine). A treatment is considered *symptomatic* if it temporarily helps symptoms but doesn't actually cure or modify the course of the underlying disease. For example, a symptomatic treatment for pneumonia would be aspirin because it provides temporary relief. However, to cure pneumonia, the patient would need to take an antibiotic, which would be a disease-modifying treatment.

If you do decide to volunteer for a clinical trial, keep in mind that the intervention is still being investigated and not yet proven to be effective. Many people who volunteer for these studies have unrealistic expectations and believe that a new and innovative approach will definitely eliminate their own disease. Also, most of these clinical trials include placebo groups, so there is always a chance that the volunteer will not be receiving an active treatment.

In addition to helping society find better Alzheimer's treatments, volunteering for a clinical trial can have several benefits for the participant. The treatment may be effective, which means that the volunteers who receive the active drug may be the first to benefit from it. The medical assessments required for enrollment may also detect an otherwise unknown medical illness that can then be treated.

If you or a loved one is considering a clinical trial, it's important to determine if you can continue to take your approved Alzheimer's treatment while enrolled in the trial. Clinical trial research is essential for moving us closer to better treatments, but it's also very important that patient volunteers receive the current standard of care while enrolled in a study.

CHECKLIST WHEN CONSIDERING ENROLLMENT IN A CLINICAL TRIAL

☐ Are you comfortable with the potential risks?

☐ Is the study team reputable?

☐ Have they reviewed the informed consent form with you and answered all of your questions?

☐ What is the likelihood you will be given a placebo?

☐ If the treatment works, how much benefit can you expect?

☐ Will you be able to continue your current treatments for Alzheimer's and your other medical conditions?

☐ Is the time commitment feasible for you?

☐ Is there a requirement for a study partner to accompany you to appointments?

During the past decade, researchers have focused their studies on earlier stages of the disease. This strategy is based on the idea that protecting healthy brain cells will be more efficient than attempting to repair a brain that is already extensively damaged from disease. That means that you may enroll in a clinical trial even if you only have mild symptoms for which symptomatic drugs are not yet indicated.

Families and patients interested in participating in the studies can go online to www.clinicaltrials.gov

and search for Alzheimer's disease. Another resource is the Alzheimer's Association (www.alz.org), which provides additional opportunities and resources.

RESEARCH ON DISEASE BIOMARKERS

Even though doctors and scientists have improved their ability to identify who has Alzheimer's disease and who does not, accuracy of clinical diagnosis is not 100 percent. This creates a problem for clinical researchers because they may be testing a new anti-Alzheimer's drug in some volunteers who don't have the disease. To address this issue, scientists have developed brain scans and other diagnostic tools to improve their accuracy in pinpointing the extent of the disease in living people.

Although these tools are helpful in improving diagnostic accuracy in clinical trials, they can be misleading for patients and families. A lot of the work in this area is focused on developing brain positron emission tomography (PET) scans that can provide a visualization of the amyloid plaques and tau tangles in the brains of living people. Until the development of this technology, these abnormal proteins could only be observed under the microscope in autopsied brain tissue obtained after the patient's death. Although the FDA has approved some of the new amyloid PET scans, the Centers for Medicare and

Medicaid Services have not yet determined that these scans provide added value to patients in clinical settings, so Medicare and other insurance carriers will currently not pay for them. Keep in mind that some people who receive a positive amyloid scan will never develop Alzheimer's dementia in their lifetime, while others with negative scans may eventually develop the disease.

In my practice I've seen several individuals who were experiencing only mild memory complaints and yet decided to get an amyloid PET scan. Although these scans are not always predictive of an Alzheimer's diagnosis, people whose amyloid scans come back positive tend to develop considerable anxiety about their cognitive abilities declining.

Some research has shown that people who discover they are carriers of the APOE-4 genetic risk for Alzheimer's disease perform worse on memory tests compared with their counterparts who were not informed of their genetic risk status. This suggests that knowledge of an abnormal test result can cause heightened anxiety that worsens memory performance. Other research suggests that knowledge of a person's own genetic risk can sometimes motivate them to live a healthier lifestyle in order to offset that genetic risk. When considering volunteering for a research study, keep in mind the potential risks and benefits of knowing about your disease-risk status.

Although brain scan research is promising, these procedures can be expensive. An alternative approach, lumbar puncture, can be done to check levels of abnormal amyloid and tau proteins in the cerebral spinal fluid. However, many people are uncomfortable with the idea of the lumbar puncture procedure, which may cause headaches and, rarely, infections. As a result, scientists are searching for inexpensive, noninvasive biomarker tests. One potentially promising approach is a sniff test that attempts to identify people in the early stages of Alzheimer's disease by testing their ability to recognize fragrances. For now, most of these biomarkers are still in the investigative stages and not ready for actual clinical use.

EXAMPLES OF BIOMARKERS UNDER STUDY FOR ALZHEIMER'S DISEASE

- *Blood tests*. Genetic tests (apoliprotein E, presenilin, and amyloid precursor protein mutations), amyloid, tau

- *Cerebrospinal fluid tests*. Amyloid beta-42, phosphorylated tau

- *Brain scanning*. Magnetic resonance imaging (MRI) scans of regional brain volumes, diffusion tensor imaging (DTI) of white matter, functional MRI regional neural activation, electroencephalography (EEG), single photon emission tomography (SPECT), PET of amyloid and/or tau

- *Other strategies.* Sniff test, head size, vascular risk factors (e.g., cholesterol levels)

DIFFERENT STRATEGIES FOR ATTACKING THE DISEASE

Amyloid plaques have been shown to be toxic to brain cells in experimental laboratories, but some research suggests that these protein deposits may actually be a response to some other abnormal process that is causing the disease. For example, when scientists study amyloid plaques under the microscope, they find evidence of inflammation. Therefore, it is possible that plaque formation in the brain is a response to brain inflammation rather than being an underlying cause of the disease.

I believe that it is important for investigators to diversify their disease targets because we now know that several different abnormal mechanisms contribute to Alzheimer's disease. In addition to the accumulation of insoluble amyloid plaques and tau tangles in the brains of patients with the disease, we also know that inflammatory responses are damaging normal cells, brain cells are misfiring, and blood circulation to brain cells is compromised.

Considerable evidence points to the contribution of heightened inflammation as a driving force behind Alzheimer's disease. In the 1990s, the Baltimore Longitudinal Study of Aging showed that older adults who took anti-inflammatory medicines for two or more years had a 60 percent lower rate of developing the disease. Interestingly, investigators then tested these medicines in patients who already had Alzheimer's dementia and found that they did not work at that stage of the disease.

EXAMPLES OF ALZHEIMER'S TREATMENTS UNDER STUDY

- Antibodies, pills, and vaccines against abnormal amyloid and tau brain proteins
- Diabetes and cholesterol-lowering medicines
- Behavioral interventions (e.g., cognitive training, healthy lifestyle regimens)
- Dietary supplements (e.g., curcumin, omega-3 fats, pomegranate extract, resveratrol)
- Neuromodulation (e.g., low-frequency focused ultrasound, deep brain stimulation, electromagnetic devices)
- Stem cell infusions

Other research shows that anti-inflammatory strategies used earlier in the course of neurodegeneration may benefit cognitive abilities and improve brain function. Our UCLA group studied people with normal aging or mild cognitive impairment over an 18-month period and discovered cognitive benefits from anti-inflammatory treatments. Because this study included a relatively small sample size and anti-inflammatory medicines have many side effects, we continued to search for less toxic strategies to reduce inflammation in people at risk for dementia. Our initial studies using the anti-inflammatory spice curcumin and pomegranate juice showed that they may offer cognitive benefits when consumed daily. Other research confirming the benefits of physical exercise support this anti-inflammatory hypothesis because cardiovascular conditioning is known to reduce inflammation.

Due to the fact that diabetes increases the risk for developing Alzheimer's dementia, some investigators are testing nasal insulin sprays or diabetes medicines like metformin. Estrogen, testosterone and other hormones are also being tested as possible treatments.

Other lines of research have used a variety of technologies to improve brain function. Some scientists are focusing ultrasound waves on the brain's hippocampal memory center in attempts to jumpstart cognitive neural circuits. Magnets, electrical currents, and other neuromodulation methods are also under development and show promise for the future.

To definitely show that a treatment works, it must be compared to a sham or placebo treatment in people suffering from the disease at various stages. These studies take many years to complete, and even before interventions can be tested in humans, they must be shown to be safe and effective in animals in the laboratory. Patients and families often hear about early results in the laboratory and mistakenly assume that a novel intervention is safe and effective for humans. However, just because an intervention works in the laboratory or in animals, it doesn't prove that it will be safe and effective in people.

CHAPTER 8

Planning for the Future

*If you don't know where you are
going, you'll end up someplace else.*
—Yogi Berra

ACCORDING TO THE FRENCH proverb, the more things change, the more they stay the same. Caring for a patient with Alzheimer's disease or another type of dementia involves adapting to constant changes and the escalating needs of the patient. Many families find that as soon as they adjust to a loved one's level of cognitive decline and behavioral disturbances, a new problem pops up that must be addressed. This sad reality of the disease is important for caregivers to be aware of and accept. Anticipating some of the future challenges of caregiving can lower caregiver stress and reduce their burden of care.

WHEN DOES GENETIC TESTING MAKE SENSE?

Planning for the future may involve learning about one's genetic risk. We know that genetic risk has an impact on if and when someone develops Alzheimer's dementia. For the average person, genetics account for less than half the risk, but it still remains a concern for many families. Children and grandchildren of dementia patients often want to know whether they will eventually develop the disease.

When discussions about genetics and family history come up in my practice, I let people know that although having a parent with Alzheimer's doubles an adult child's risk for getting the disease, it is far from a sure thing.

Families with genetic risks for dementia fall into two types: families where only occasional relatives are affected, and families where half of all relatives are affected. The families where half of relatives are affected by the disease have what geneticists call an autosomal dominant inheritance pattern. This means that a genetic defect or mutation for the disease is transmitted from generation to generation. Someone from such a family has a 50 percent risk of developing Alzheimer's dementia.

These families are quite rare, but anyone from such a family might wish to consult with a genetic counselor to review the pros and cons of learning of their genetic profile. One of the positives, of course, is having a more realistic expectation for the future and being able to plan ahead. However, emotional reactions to the knowledge of genetic information can vary. Some people who learn they have a genetic mutation for the disease become depressed about their future. On occasion, family members who discover that they do not have the mutation can become depressed as well, usually because of survival guilt that comes from knowing other close family members do have the genetic mutation.

For the vast majority of people, having a genetic mutation that causes the disease is not a relevant issue. However, there are concerns about certain genetic risks for the disease, such as APOE-4, which affects 20 percent of the population. Being an APOE-4 carrier increases one's chances of developing dementia at an earlier age, but it is not an absolute outcome. I don't routinely recommend testing for these genetic risks because learning of them can cause anxiety in many people. For some patients, however, it can motivate them to live a healthier lifestyle in order to offset their genetic risk.

ADVANCED DIRECTIVES

Advance directives are legal documents indicating an individual's future wishes regarding their health care, finances, and other matters in case they no longer have the capacity to make such decisions in the future. They also include designations of who will be making those decisions for them. These documents are drawn up and signed while the person still has decision-making capacity. Without advance directives in place, family members will have to make these decisions for the patient, and those decisions may not be consistent with what the patient would have wanted. Commonly used advance directives include:

- *Living will.* Establishes a person's desires about end-of-life care (e.g., types of treatments, use of life-support systems)
- *Durable power of attorney for healthcare.* Assigns medical decision-making authority to a particular person
- *Estate will.* Describes how to deal with the person's property after death

Just because someone has a diagnosis of Alzheimer's dementia does not necessarily mean that they no longer have capacity to make decisions about their finances, health care, or other important matters. A patient with dementia may be unable to drive but may still have the capacity to handle their financial affairs or live independently. Sometimes families will appoint a legal guardian for specific tasks such as financial management but may still permit the patient to have control over other matters.

Once you have advanced directives in place, make sure that you distribute copies of the documents to all of those involved, and ensure that they understand the directives. Sometimes family members disagree on some aspects of the directives, and it is best to try to resolve such conflicts while the patient can still be involved in the discussions.

STRATEGIES FOR DEALING WITH CONFLICTS OVER ADVANCED DIRECTIVES

- *Listen.* Respect each family member's opinion about end-of-life preferences and quality of care.

- *Avoid blame.* This is a typical response that only escalates conflict.

- *Share feelings.* Candidly discussing each person's concerns and fears can be helpful in breaking through destructive denial about the illness and help resolve disagreements.

- *Involve a third party.* A therapist, mediator, doctor, spiritual leader, or any third party everyone trusts can help smooth over difficult issues.

- *Get support.* Conflicts often stem from differing emotional reactions that can lead to inefficient coping skills. The Alzheimer's Association's support groups can help your family work through the many emotions that emerge, including guilt, depression, grief, and anger.

These discussions will be fruitful if those involved are able to review the details of the directives. For example, health-care issues to consider will include the use of antibiotics for infections; artificial nutrition or nutrients provided via a tube into the stomach, intestine, or vein; do not resuscitate orders (instructions not to perform cardiopulmonary resuscitation [CPR] if the heart or breathing stops); ventilator machines; and more.

Assisted suicide is a controversial issue, especially for patients with dementia. David Goodall, a 104-year-old Australian scientist, was aware of his diminishing cognitive and visual capacities and knew he would eventually need 24-hour care. Because euthanasia is illegal in his country, he flew to Switzerland, where a euthanasia advocacy group assisted him with his suicide.

Although some US states allow physician-assisted suicide, there are many restrictions regarding the presence of a terminal illness leading to death in a defined time period and demonstrating that the person who chooses assisted suicide is mentally competent. This last restriction can be a major obstacle for patients with dementia. Anyone interested in exploring this issue in more detail should consult with an attorney who specializes in elder care and related issues.

MANAGING FINANCES

Some older adults who are developing dementia have no problem letting their spouses or adult children take over control of their finances. They often work with their attorneys and appoint the appropriate loved ones as cotrustees of their estates.

In other families, it is not so easy. A parent developing dementia may be reluctant to accept help from others. Some patients with MCI or mild Alzheimer's insist on writing their own checks for the household and for gifts to extended family members. Sometimes financial mishaps can occur, and family members have to step in. These mishaps can include unpaid bills, bounced checks, and irregular spending.

Many older adults fall for the "grandparents scam," wherein someone claiming to work at the US embassy in a foreign country phones to say that their grandchild is in jail or in some kind of trouble. The scammer demands money for the grandchild's release, and the older adult ends up wiring thousands of dollars to the con artist.

Money carries a lot of emotional power for older parents and their adult children. Many caring parents want to express their love to their kids through gifts. Others may use money to control their children's lives. Monetary resources help us take charge of our lives, and when aging parents need to trust others with their finances, they are forced to give up some or all of that control.

TIPS ON MANAGING MONEY FOR A LOVED ONE WITH DEMENTIA

- Consult with an attorney and financial planner in advance so your loved one can have input on future plans

- Watch for warning signs of financial issues:
  - Trouble determining change for a purchase
  - Difficulty balancing a checkbook
  - Forgetting to pay bills
  - Unusual credit card charges

- If your loved one is unable to manage their money, you can put safeguards in place to protect them:
  - Add a cosigner to their bank accounts
  - Automate bill paying if possible
  - Provide only a small amount of money for their wallet or purse
  - Limit credit card access
  - Routinely review credit reports

The transfer of wealth to younger generations also stirs up sibling rivalries. I've seen many families torn apart by battles over wills and trusts. For some families, it is almost impossible to separate emotions from financial planning. However, there are strategies to help recognize when a cognitively impaired family member needs help as well as ways that safeguards can be put in place.

An important aspect of financial planning involves health-care insurance. Older adults are eligible for Medicare. Part A covers hospital stays, while part B covers physician services and outpatient care. For outpatient prescription drug coverage, a separate part D prescription policy is required. Medicare Advantage plans offer medication and medical coverage through private insurance.

Medicaid provides health coverage for some low-income older adults and can provide secondary insurance, including long-term care. Long-term care insurance policies can assist with costs of care for chronic medical conditions such as Alzheimer's disease. Most policies offer reimbursement for care provided in different settings, such as the patient's or caregiver's home, an assisted living facility, or a nursing home.

SENIOR LIVING OPTIONS

As a loved one's cognitive challenges progress, family members must decide on the safest and best living option. Many older adults are reluctant to move from their homes because of fear that they will be put out to pasture in a substandard nursing facility. However, many comfortable and lovely living options are available. In my practice, I often see widows who insist on remaining in their homes, isolated from friends and family. Unfortunately, such isolation further accelerates cognitive decline. I often encourage these elders to move to a senior living setting where there are opportunities for social interaction and greater mental stimulation.

Many factors weigh into the decision about the best living setting, particularly the patient's finances and daily care needs. The following are some options to consider:

- *Staying home.* If your loved one remains relatively independent, this may be the best option. Caregivers can be hired to help with meals, cleaning, daily chores, and activities.
- *Independent living.* These housing options are designed exclusively for older adults and include retirement communities, senior housing, and senior apartments. These communities offer maintenance services, meals, housekeeping, and group activities.
- *Residential care homes.* These facilities (e.g., adult family homes, board and care homes) provide personalized services to small groups

of adults, including meals and assistance with daily activities.

- *Assisted living.* Older adults who can still live independently but need greater assistance can receive 24-hour care and help with medication management, bathing, dressing, housekeeping, and transportation. They also have group dining and common areas for socializing.

- *Nursing homes or skilled nursing facilities.* These settings are for older adults in need of 24-hour supervised care and include meals, activities, and health management. A nurse or other health-care professional remains on site, and a physician supervises each resident's care. Some facilities provide specialized Alzheimer's care.

- *Continuing care retirement communities.* These facilities offer different levels of care depending on the resident's needs and typically include independent living, assisted living, and skilled nursing areas. This kind of setting suits the needs of older adults who want to live in one location for the rest of their lives. They work well for spouses who want to stay close to one another even if one partner needs more care than the other.

LOOKING TO THE FUTURE WHILE APPRECIATING THE PRESENT

Patients with Alzheimer's disease and their families face a daunting journey with many uncertainties, ups and downs, and eventual steady worsening of the patient's health. Anticipating those future vicissitudes does help lower the burden of the disease, but it is important to enjoy and be grateful for the present while the patient's cognitive abilities are still relatively intact. Some caregivers and family members are so focused on future anticipated problems that they fail to celebrate the time they have with their loved ones while they still have the cognitive abilities to connect and appreciate each other's company.

When everyone involved tries to make the most of their available resources and acknowledges the limitations in halting Alzheimer's disease with today's tools, there is a sense of accomplishment and resolve because everything that can be done has been done. That is the most anyone can do as we await current and future research that will one day eradicate this disease and help us all live better and longer with our cognitive abilities intact.

Acknowledgments

WE APPRECIATE THE MANY patients and volunteers who have participated in the research studies that contributed to this book. Without the insights, dedication, and ingenuity of numerous colleagues, doctors, scientists, and staff at UCLA and other major research and clinical centers, this book would not have been possible. We are also thankful to our longtime agent and good friend Sandra Dijkstra, who has encouraged our writing over the years, and our publisher, Mary Glenn at Humanix Books. Finally, a special thanks to our friends, including Diana Jacobs for her drawing of the brain, and our family for their love and support, especially our children, Rachel and Harry.

Gary Small and Gigi Vorgan

Bibliography

CHAPTER 1: IS IT NORMAL AGING
OR SOMETHING WORSE?

Roose, S. P., Devanand, D., Hamilton, R., Krishnan, K. R. R., Mayeux, R., and Small, G. W. "Cognitive Impairment Associated with Depression in the Elderly." *J Clin Psychiatry* 8 (2007): 1601–12.

Small, G. W. "Detection and Prevention of Cognitive Decline." *Am J Geriatr Psychiatry* 24 (2016): 1142–50.

Small, G. W. "Differential Diagnoses and Assessment of Depression in Elderly Patients." *J Clin Psychiatry* 70 (2009): e47.

Small G. W., and Chen, S. T. "Alzheimer's Disease and Other Dementing Disorders." In *Kaplan & Sadock's Comprehensive Textbook of Psychiatry*, 10th ed., edited by B. J. Sadock, V. A. Sadock, and

P. Ruiz, 4078–86. Philadelphia, PA: Wolters Kluwer, 2017.

Small, G. W., and Jarvik, L. F. "The Dementia Syndrome." *Lancet* 2 (1982): 1443–46.

CHAPTER 2: SEEING THE DOCTOR

Coupland, C. A. C., Hill, T., Dening, T. et al. "Anticholinergic Drug Exposure and the Risk of Dementia: A Nested Case-Control Study." *JAMA Intern Med* (Jun. 24, 2019). DOI: 10.1001/jamainternmed.2019.0677.

Grossberg, G. T., Christensen, D. D., Griffith, P. A. et al. "The Art of Sharing the Diagnosis and Management of Alzheimer's Disease with Patients and Caregivers: Recommendations of an Expert Consensus Panel." *Prim Care Companion J Clin Psychiatry* 12, no. 1 (2010): PCC.09cs00833.

Knopman, D., Donohue, J. A., and Gutterman, E. M. "Patterns of Care in the Early Stages of Alzheimer's Disease: Impediments to Timely Diagnosis." *J Am Geriatr Soc* 48 (2000): 300–304.

Levenson, R. W., Sturm, V. E., and Haase, C. M. "Emotional and Behavioral Symptoms in Neurodegenerative Disease: A Model for Studying the Neural Bases of Psychopathology." *Annu Rev Clin Psychol* 10 (2010): 581–606.

Milby, E., Murphy, G., and Winthrop, A. "Diagnosis Disclosure in Dementia: Understanding the Experiences of Clinicians and Patients Who Have Recently Given or Received a Diagnosis." *Dementia* (London) 16 (2017): 611–28.

Moore, A. R., and O'Keefe, S. T. "Drug-Induced Cognitive Impairment in the Elderly." *Drugs Aging* 15 (1999): 15–28.

Small, G. W., and Chen, S. T. "Alzheimer's Disease and Other Dementing Disorders." In *Kaplan & Sadock's Comprehensive Textbook of Psychiatry*, 10th ed., edited by B. J. Sadock, V. A. Sadock, and P. Ruiz, 4078–86. Philadelphia, PA: Wolters Kluwer, 2017.

CHAPTER 3: THE LATEST ON MEDICINES AND SUPPLEMENTS

Gestuvo, M. K., and Hung, W. W. "Common Dietary Supplements for Cognitive Health." *Aging Health* 8 (2012): 89–97.

Global Council on Brain Health. "The Real Deal on Brain Health Supplements: GCBH Recommendations on Vitamins, Minerals, and Other Dietary Supplements." 2019. Available at www.GlobalCouncilOnBrainHealth.org. DOI: https://doi.org/10.26419/pia.00094.001.

O'Brien, J. T., Holmes, C., Jones, M. et al. "Clinical Practice with Anti-dementia Drugs." *J Psychopharmacol* 31 (2017): 147–68.

Rabins, P. V., Graff-Radford, N., Small, G. W., and Yaari, R. "New Developments in the Treatment of Alzheimer's Disease." *J Clin Psychiatry* 70 (2009): 281–90.

Rao, V., and Lyketso, C. G. "The Benefits and Risks of ECT for Patients with Primary Dementia Who Also Suffer from Depression." *Int J Geriatr Psychiatry* 15 (2000): 729–35.

Shineman, D. W., Salthouse, T. A., Launer, L. J. et al. "Therapeutics for Cognitive Aging." *Ann New York Acad Sci* 1191 (Suppl 1, 2010): E1–15.

Small, G., and Bullock R. "Defining Optimal Treatment with Cholinesterase Inhibitors in Alzheimer's Disease." *Alzheimer's Dementia* 7 (2011): 177–84.

Small G. W., Siddarth P., Li, Z. et al. "Memory and Brain Amyloid and Tau Effects of a Bioavailable Form of Curcumin in Non-demented Adults: A Double-Blind, Placebo-Controlled 18-Month Trial." *Am J Geriatr Psychiatry* 26 (2018): 266–77.

CHAPTER 4: PRACTICAL STRATEGIES FOR CAREGIVERS

Allan, L. M., Ballard, C. G., Rowan, E. N., and Kenny R. A. "Incidence and Prediction of Falls in Dementia:

A Prospective Study in Older People." *PLOS One* 4, no. 5 (2009): e5521.

Brown, L. B, and Ott, B. R. "Driving and Dementia: A Review of the Literature." *J Geriatr Psychiatry Neurol* 17 (2004): 232–40.

Cheng, S.-T. "Dementia Caregiver Burden: A Research Update and Critical Analysis." *Curr Psychiatry Rep* 19 (2017): 64.

Pew Research Center. "Seniors and Technology." Available at https://www.pewinternet.org/2017/05/17/technology-use-among-seniors/.

Steptoe, A., Deaton, A., and Stone, A. A. "Psychological Wellbeing, Health and Ageing." *Lancet* 385 (2015): 640–48.

CHAPTER 5: THE EMOTIONAL ROLLER COASTER OF CAREGIVING

Barger, S. D. "Social Integration, Social Support and Mortality in the US National Health Interview Survey." *Psychosom Med* 75 (2013): 510–17.

Carney, C. E., Edinger, J. D., Kuchibhatla, M. et al. "Cognitive Behavioral Insomnia Therapy for Those with Insomnia and Depression: A Randomized Controlled Clinical Trial." *Sleep* 40, no. 4 (Apr. 1, 2017). DOI: 10.1093/sleep/zsx019.

Cheng, S. T. "Dementia Caregiver Burden: A Research Update and Critical Analysis." *Curr Psychiatry*

Rep 19, no. 9 (Aug. 10, 2017): 64. DOI: 10.1007/
s11920-017-0818-2.

Damjanovic, A. K., Yang, Y., Glaser, R. et al. "Accelerated Telomere Erosion Is Associated with a
Declining Immune Function of Caregivers of Alzheimer's Disease Patients." *J Immunol* 179 (2007):
4249–54.

Khondoker, M., Rafnsson, S. G., Morris, S. et al. "Positive and Negative Experiences of Social Support
and Risk of Dementia in Later Life: An Investigation Using the English Longitudinal Study of Ageing." *J Alzheimer's Dis* 58 (2017): 99–108.

Kvam, S., Kleppe, C. L., Nordhus, I. H., and Hovland,
A. "Exercise as a Treatment for Depression: A
Meta-analysis." *J Affect Disord* 202 (Sep. 15, 2016):
67–86.

McEwen, B. S. "Central Effects of Stress Hormones in
Health and Disease: Understanding the Protective
and Damaging Effects of Stress and Stress Media-
tors." *Eur J Pharmacol* 583 (2008): 174–85.

Sutin, A. R., Stephan, Y., Luchetti, M. et al. "Loneliness
and Risk of Dementia." *J Gerontol B Psychol Sci Soc
Sci* (Oct. 26, 2018). DOI: 10.1093/geronb/gby112.

Vandepitte, S., Putman, K., Van Den Noorgate, N. et
al. "Effectiveness of an In-Home Respite Care Program to Support Informal Dementia Caregivers: A
Comparative Study." *J Geriatr Psychiatry* (Jun. 26,
2019). DOI: 10.1002/gps.5164.

CHAPTER 6: LIFESTYLE HABITS
THAT PROTECT YOUR BRAIN

Anguera, J. A., Boccanfuso, J., Rintoul, J. L. et al. "Video Game Training Enhances Cognitive Control in Older Adults." *Nature* 501 (Sep. 5, 2013): 97–101.

Anstey, K. J., Mack, H. A., and Cherbuin, N. "Alcohol Consumption as a Risk Factor for Dementia and Cognitive Decline: Meta-analysis of Prospective Studies." *Am J Geriatr Psychiatry* 17 (2009): 542–55.

Barnes, D. E., and Yaffe, K. "The Projected Effect of Risk Factor Reduction on Alzheimer's Disease Prevalence." *Lancet Neurol* 10 (2011): 819–28.

Bookheimer, S. Y., Renner, B. A., Ekstrom, A. et al. "Pomegranate Juice Augments Memory and fMRI Activity in Middle-Aged and Older Adults with Mild Memory Complaints." *Evid Based Complement Alternat Med* 2013 (2013): 946298. DOI: 10.1155/2013/946298.

Borella, E., Carretti, B., Zanoni, G. et al. "Working Memory Training in Old Age: An Examination of Transfer and Maintenance Effects." *Arch Clin Neuropsychol* 28 (2013): 331–47.

Chen, S. T., Siddarth, P., Ercoli, L. M. et al. "Modifiable Risk Factors for Alzheimer Disease and Subjective Memory Impairment across Age Groups." *PLOS*

One 9, no. 6 (June 4, 2014): e98630. DOI: 10.1371/ journal.pone.0098630. eCollection 2014.

Debette, S., Beiser, A., Hoffmann, U. et al. "Visceral Fat Is Associated with Lower Brain Volume in Healthy Middle-Aged Adults." *Ann Neurol* 68 (2010): 136–44.

Erickson, K. I., Voss, M. W., Prakash, R. S. et al. "Exercise Training Increases Size of Hippocampus and Improves Memory." *Proc Natl Acad Sci USA* 108 (2010): 3017–22.

Eskelinen, M. H., and Kivipelto, M. "Caffeine as a Protective Factor in Dementia and Alzheimer's Disease." *J Alzheimer's Dis* 20, suppl. 1 (2010): S167–74.

Fitzpatrick, A. L., Kuller, L. H., Lopez, O. L. et al. "Midlife and Late-Life Obesity and the Risk of Dementia: Cardiovascular Health Study." *Arch Neurol* 66 (2009): 336–42.

Graafland, M., Bemelman, W. A., and Schijven, M. P. "Game-Based Training Improves the Surgeon's Situational Awareness in the Operation Room: A Randomized Controlled Trial." *Surg Endosc* 31 (2017): 4093–101.

Heyn, P., Abreu, B. C., and Ottenbacher, K. J. "The Effects of Exercise Training on Elderly Persons with Cognitive Impairment and Dementia: A Meta-analysis." *Arch Phys Med Rehab* 85 (2004): 1694–1704.

Merrill, D. A., and Small, G. W. "Prevention in Psychiatry: Effects of Healthy Lifestyle on Cognition." *Psychiatr Clin N Amer* 34 (2011): 249–61.

Miller, K. J., Dye, R. V., Kim, J. et al. "Effect of a Computerized Brain Exercise Program on Cognitive Performance in Older Adults." *Am J Geriatr Psychiatry* 21 (2013): 655–63.

Neuhoff, C. C., and Schaefer, C. "Effects of Laughing, Smiling, and Howling on Mood." *Psychol Rep* 91 (2002): 1079–80.

Rebok, G. W., Ball, K., Guey, L. T. et al. "Ten-Year Effects of the Advanced Cognitive Training for Independent and Vital Elderly Cognitive Training Trial on Cognition and Everyday Functioning in Older Adults." *J Am Geriatr Soc* 62 (2014): 16–24.

Rosenberg, A., Ngandu, T., and Rusanen, M. "Multidomain Lifestyle Intervention Benefits a Large Elderly Population at Risk for Cognitive Decline and Dementia Regardless of Baseline Characteristics: The FINGER Trial." *Alzheimer's Dementia* 14 (2018): 263–70.

Siddarth, P., Li, Z., Miller, K. J. et al. "Randomized Placebo-Controlled Study of the Memory Effects of Pomegranate Juice in Middle-Aged and Older Adults." *Am J Clin Nutr* 2019 Nov 12. pii: nqz241. doi: 10.1093/ajcn/nqz241.

Small, G. W., Moody, T. D., Siddarth, P., and Bookheimer, S. Y. "Your Brain on Google: Patterns of Cerebral Activation during Internet Searching." *Am J Geriatr Psychiatry* 17 (2009): 116–26.

Small, G. W., Siddarth, P., Ercoli, L. M. et al. "Healthy Behavior and Memory Self-Reports in Young,

Middle-Aged, and Older Adults." *Int Psychogeri-atr* 25 (2013): 981–89.

Small, G. W., Siddarth, P., Li, Z. et al. "Memory and Brain Amyloid and Tau Effects of a Bioavailable Form of Curcumin in Non-demented Adults: A Double-Blind, Placebo-Controlled 18-Month Trial." *Am J Geriatr Psychiatry* 26 (2018): 266–77.

Small, G. W., Silverman, D. H., Siddarth, P. et al. "Effects of a 14-Day Healthy Longevity Lifestyle Program on Cognition and Brain Function." *Am J Geriatr Psychiatry* 14 (2006): 538–45.

Spira, A. P., Gamaldo, A. A., An, Y. et al. "Self-Reported Sleep and β-Amyloid Deposition in Community-Dwelling Older Adults." *JAMA Neurol* 70 (2013): 1537–43.

Weinstein, G., Beiser, A. S., Choi, S. H. et al. "Serum Brain-Derived Neurotrophic Factor and the Risk for Dementia: The Framingham Heart Study." *JAMA Neurol* 71 (2014): 55–61.

World Health Organization. "Obesity and Overweight." Available at http://www.who.int/dietphysicalactivity/media/en/gsfs_obesity.pdf.

Ybarra, O., Burnstein, E., Winkielman, P. et al. "Mental Exercising through Simple Socializing: Social Interaction Promotes General Cognitive Functioning." *Pers Soc Psychol Bull* 34 (2008): 248–59.

CHAPTER 7: NEW RESEARCH: HYPE VS. HOPE

Bookheimer, S. Y., Renner, B. A., Ekstrom, A. et al. "Pomegranate Juice Augments Memory and fMRI Activity in Middle-Aged and Older Adults with Mild Memory Complaints." *Evid Based Complement Alternat Med* 2013 (2013): 946298. DOI: 10.1155/2013/946298.

Cummings, J., Lee, G., Ritter, A., Sabbagh, M., and Zhong, K. "Alzheimer's Disease Drug Development Pipeline: 2019." *Alzheimer's & Dementia: Journal of the Alzheimer's Association* 5 (July 9, 2019): 272–93. DOI: 10.1016/j.trci.2019.05.008. eCollection 2019.

Green, R. C., Roberts, J. S., Cupples, L. A. et al. "Disclosure of APOE Genotype for Risk of Alzheimer's Disease." *N Engl J Med* 361 (2009): 245–54.

Hietaranta-Luoma, H. L., Tringham, M., Karjalainen, H. et al. "A Long-Term Follow-Up Study on Disclosing Genetic Risk Information (APOE) to Promote Healthy Lifestyles in Finland." *Lifestyle Genom* 11 (2018): 147–54.

McEwen, S. C., Siddarth, P., Abedelsater, B. et al. "Simultaneous Aerobic Exercise and Memory Training Program in Older Adults with Subjective Memory Impairments." *J Alzheim Dis* 62 (2018): 795–806.

Sharma, N., and Nikita Singh, A. "Exploring Biomarkers for Alzheimer's Disease." *J Clin Diagn Res* 10, no. 7 (July 2016): KE01–KE06. DOI: 10.7860/JCDR/2016/18828.8166.

Siddarth, P., Li, Z., Miller, K. J. et al. "Randomized Placebo-Controlled Study of the Memory Effects of Pomegranate Juice in Middle-Aged and Older Adults." *Am J Clin Nutr* 2019 Nov 12. pii: nqz241. doi: 10.1093/ajcn/nqz241.

Siddarth, P., Rahi, B., Emerson, N. D. et al. "Physical Activity and Hippocampal Sub-region Structure in Older Adults with Memory Complaints." *J Alzheim Dis* 61 (2018): 1089–96.

Small, G. W., Bookheimer, S. Y., Thompson, P. M. et al. "Current and Future Uses of Neuroimaging for Cognitively Impaired Patients." *Lancet Neurol* 7 (2008): 161–72.

Small, G. W., Siddarth, P., Li, Z. et al. "Memory and Brain Amyloid and Tau Effects of a Bioavailable Form of Curcumin in Non-demented Adults: A Double-Blind, Placebo-Controlled 18-Month Trial." *Am J Geriatr Psychiatry* 26 (2018): 266–77.

Small, G. W., Siddarth, P., Silverman, D. H. S. et al. "Cognitive and Cerebral Metabolic Effects of Celecoxib versus Placebo in People with Age-Related Memory Loss: Randomized Controlled Study." *Am J Geriatr Psychiatry* 16 (2008): 999–1009.

Stewart, W. F., Kawas, C., Corrada, M., and Metter, E. J. "Risk of Alzheimer's Disease and Duration and I Are of NSAID Use." *Neurology* 48 (1997): 626–32.

CHAPTER 8: PLANNING FOR THE FUTURE

Davis, D. S. "Advance Directives and Alzheimer's Disease." *J Law Med Ethics* 46 (2018): 744–48.

Goldman, J. S, Hahn, S. E., Catania, J. W. et al. "Genetic Counseling and Testing for Alzheimer Disease: Joint Practice Guidelines of the American College of Medical Genetics and the National Society of Genetic Counselors." *Genet Med* 13 (2011): 597–605.

Joseph, Y., and Magra, I. "David Goodall, 104, Scientist Who Fought to Die on His Terms, Ends His Life." *New York Times* (May 10, 2018).

Mace, N. L., and Rabins, P. V. *The 36-Hour Day*. New York: Warner Books, 1999.

Reisenwitz, T. H. "Exploring Senior Living Alternatives to Institutional Care: Differences between Residents and Non-residents." *Global Business Review* (Apr. 30, 2017). Available at https://doi.org/10.1177/0972150917693153.

Sudo, F. K., and Laks, J. "Financial Capacity in Dementia: A Systematic Review." *Aging Ment Health* 21 (2017): 677–83.

Index

Page numbers in *italics* refer to figures.

About the Authors

Dr. Gary Small is a professor of psychiatry and the director of the UCLA Longevity Center at the Semel Institute for Neuroscience and Human Behavior. His research, supported by the NIH and major foundations, has made headlines in the *Wall Street Journal* and *The New York Times*. *Scientific American* magazine named him as one of the world's leading innovators in science and technology. Dr. Small lectures internationally and has often appeared on *Today*, *Good Morning America*, PBS, and CNN. He has written 10 books, including the *New York Times* bestseller *The Memory Bible*.

Gigi Vorgan has written, produced, and appeared in numerous feature films and television projects before teaming up with her husband, Dr. Gary Small, to cowrite *The Memory Bible*, *The Memory*

Prescription, The Longevity Bible, iBrain, The Other Side of the Couch, The Alzheimer's Prevention Program, 2 Weeks to a Younger Brain, SNAP! Change Your Personality in 30 Days, and *The Small Guide to Anxiety.*

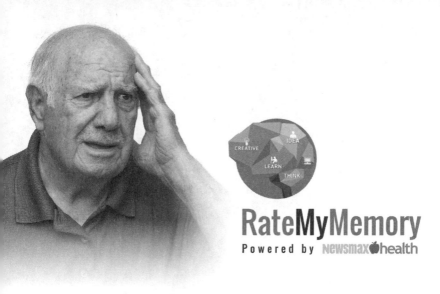

Normal Forgetfulness?
Something More Serious?

You forget things — names of people, where you parked your car, the place you put an important document, and so much more. Some experts tell you to dismiss these episodes.

"Not so fast," says Dr. Gary Small, director of the UCLA Longevity Center, medical researcher, professor of psychiatry, and the *New York Times* best-selling author of *2 Weeks to a Younger Brain.*

Dr. Small says that most age-related memory issues are normal but sometimes can be a warning sign of future cognitive decline.

Now Dr. Small has created the online **RateMyMemory Test** — allowing you to easily assess your memory strength in just a matter of minutes.

It's time to begin your journey of making sure your brain stays healthy and young! **It takes just 2 minutes!**

Test Your Memory Today:
MemoryRate.com/Small

Improve Memory and Sharpen Your Mind

Misplacing your keys, forgetting someone's name at a party, or coming home from the market without the most important item — these are just some of the many common memory slips we all experience from time to time.

Most of us laugh about these occasional memory slips, but for some, it's no joke. Are these signs of dementia, or worse, Alzheimer's? Dr. Garry Small will help dissuade those fears and teach you practical strategies and exercises to sharpen your mind in his breakthrough book, *2 Weeks To A Younger Brain*.

This book will show that it only takes two weeks to form new habits that bolster cognitive abilities and help stave off or even reverse brain aging.

If you commit only 14 days to *2 Weeks To A Younger Brain*, you will reap noticeable results. During that brief period, you will have learned the secrets of keeping your brain young for the rest of your life.

Claim Your FREE OFFER Now!

Claim your **FREE** copy of *2 Weeks To A Younger Brain* — a $19.99 value — today with this special offer. Just cover $4.95 for shipping & handling.

Plus, you will receive a 3-month risk-free trial subscription to *Dr. Gary Small's Mind Health Report*. Renowned brain expert and psychiatrist Gary Small, M.D., fills every issue of *Mind Health Report* with the latest advancements and breakthrough techniques for improving & enhancing your memory, brain health, and longevity. **That's a $29 value, yours FREE!**

More Titles From Humanix Books You May Be Interested In:

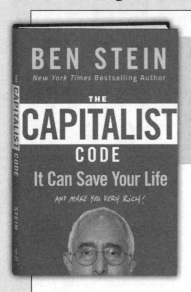

Warren Buffett says:
"My friend, Ben Stein, has written a short book that tells you everything you need to know about investing (and in words you can understand). Follow Ben's advice and you will do far better than almost all investors (and I include pension funds, universities and the super-rich) who pay high fees to advisors."

In his entertaining and informative style that has captivated generations, beloved *New York Times* bestselling author, actor, and financial expert Ben Stein sets the record straight about capitalism in the United States — it is not the "rigged system" young people are led to believe.

Dr. Mehmet Oz says:
"*SNAP!* shows that personalities can be changed from what our genes or early childhood would have ordained. Invest the 30 days."

New York Times bestselling author Dr. Gary Small's breakthrough plan to improve your personality for a better life! As you read *SNAP!* you will gain a better understanding of who you are now, how others see you, and which aspects of yourself you'd like to change. You will acquire the tools you need to change your personality in just one month — it won't take years of psychotherapy, self-exploration, or re-hashing every single bad thing that's ever happened to you.

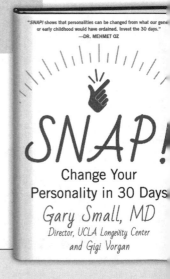

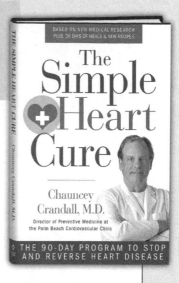